本书由复旦大学出版资助基金资助

Measuring Health-State Utilities for Cost-Utility Analysis

测量健康效用以用于成本效用分析

王 沛 著

復旦大學 出版社

Foreword

In China, the use of cost-utility analysis (CUA) which is the most frequently used economic evaluation method, has been dramatically increased in recent years. On the other hand, research on health utility, which is the kernel component of CUA, is still lacking in the context of China. Such a gap may have significantly affected the validity of CUA results and thus the decision on resource allocations in health care in China.

The book investigated several fundamental issues on health utility assessment, including whether health utility derived from other populations could be adopted directly in targeted populations; how to select different utility instruments; how to predict health utility using data from non-utility instruments; how to model observed health utility data; how to select different utility instruments, etc. I sincerely hope the results and discussions of the issues could stimulate more theoretical and empirical health utility studies based on various Chinese populations.

I would like to express my sincerest gratitude to my supervisor, Prof. Luo Nan from Saw Swee Hock School of Public Health, National University of Singapore (NUS), for his direction, patience and high standards in research. He has taught me a lot about how to do research and write academic papers. He also spent many hours reviewing my original manuscripts, gave valuable suggestions and made detailed editions. His support has been invaluable for me to complete this book.

I am also grateful to my supervisor, Prof. Julian Thumboo, and Prof. Lee Hin Peng from NUS for their continuous support, suggestions to accomplish my work. My sincere thanks also go to Assoc. Prof. Tai E Shyong from NUS, who provided research subjects for me. I am also thankful to Prof. Cheung Yin Bun from DUKE-NUS for his instructions on statistical methods. My thanks are also due to Dr. Wong Kin-Yoke for her help in questionnaire design. Many thanks go to my colleagues and office-mates, Yang Fan, Wang Xingzhi, Zhou Huijun, Chen Zhaojin, Vivian, Pan Chenwei, Jiang Jundong and Zhou Xin for their help and a source of inspiration.

Finally, I would like to deeply thank my family for their wholehearted support and continuous encouragement.

CONTENTS

Chapter 1
Introduction ········· 1
1.1 How to define health states ········· 2
1.2 How to measure HSU values ········· 3
    1.2.1 The direct method ········· 3
    1.2.2 The indirect method ········· 10
    1.2.3 Mapping health profiles to health-state utilities ········· 14
1.3 Whose health-state utilities should be used ········· 17
    1.3.1 General population health-state utilities ········· 18
    1.3.2 Patient health-state utilities ········· 19
1.4 Research objectives ········· 20
1.5 Summary of studies ········· 21

Chapter 2
Do Chinese Have Similar Health-State Preferences? A Comparison of the People in China and Chinese Singaporeans ········· 23
2.1 Introduction ········· 23
2.2 Methods ········· 25
    2.2.1 Sampling and recruitment ········· 25
    2.2.2 Procedures ········· 26
    2.2.3 EQ-VT ········· 26
    2.2.4 Health states valued ········· 28
    2.2.5 Data analysis ········· 29

Measuring Health-State Utilities for Cost-Utility Analysis
测量健康效用以用于成本效用分析

2.3 Results ·· 30
2.4 Discussion ·· 33

Chapter 3
The Impact of Diabetes on Health-State Utilities ···················· 36

3.1 Introduction ·· 36
3.2 Methods ··· 38
    3.2.1 Study participants ··· 38
    3.2.2 Survey procedures ··· 38
    3.2.3 Health states valued ··· 40
    3.2.4 Data analysis ·· 40
3.3 Results ·· 41
3.4 Discussion ·· 44

Chapter 4
Valuation of EQ-5D-3L Health States in Singapore ·················· 47

4.1 Introduction ·· 47
4.2 Methods ··· 49
    4.2.1 Sampling and recruitment ···································· 49
    4.2.2 The valuation interview ······································ 50
    4.2.3 The health states ··· 51
4.3 Statistical analysis ··· 52
    4.3.1 Calculation of TTO values ··································· 52
    4.3.2 Modeling of TTO values ····································· 52
    4.3.3 Evaluation of model performance ························· 54
4.4 Results ·· 55
    4.4.1 Respondents' characteristics ································ 55
    4.4.2 Distribution of TTO values ·································· 57
    4.4.3 Modeling analysis ··· 57
4.5 Discussion ·· 62

Chapter 5
Predicting Preference-Based SF-6D$_{36}$ Index Scores from the SF-8 Health Survey
.... 68

5.1 Introduction ·· 68
5.2 Methods ·· 69
    5.2.1 SF-8 ·· 69
    5.2.2 SF-6D$_{36}$ ·· 70
    5.2.3 Data ·· 71
    5.2.4 Model construction ·· 71
    5.2.5 Model estimation and evaluation ··································· 72
5.3 Results ·· 73
    5.3.1 Individual-level prediction ·· 74
    5.3.2 Group-level prediction ··· 78
5.4 Discussion ··· 80

Chapter 6
Preference-Based SF-6D Scores Derived from the SF-36 and SF-12 Have Different Discriminative Power in a Population Health Survey ················ 84

6.1 Introduction ·· 84
6.2 Methods ·· 85
    6.2.1 Data source ··· 85
    6.2.2 Instruments ··· 85
    6.2.3 Data analysis ··· 87
6.3 Results ·· 88
6.4 Discussion ··· 93

Chapter 7
Conclusions ··· 96

7.1 Major findings ··· 96
7.2 Contributions ··· 97

7.3　Future studies ·· 97

Chart Index ··· 99
References ·· 101

Chapter 1

Introduction

During the past three decades, cost-utility analysis (CUA) was increasingly used to inform resource allocation decisions (Torrance, 1986; Johannesson et al., 1996; Drummond et al., 2005). The CUA compares the incremental cost of a health intervention with the incremental health improvement to reflect preference attributed to the intervention. It is a form of economic appraisal method in which the health improvement is mainly measured in terms of quality-adjustment life-years (QALYs) gained (Torrance, 1986; Johannesson et al., 1996; Drummond et al., 2005). QALY incorporates both quantity and quality of life into a single generic measure by multiplying the length of life with quality-of-life weights. In the QALY approach, the quality-of-life weights are a set of health-state utilities (HSUs) (Torrance, 1986; Johannesson et al., 1996; Drummond et al., 2005). HSUs can also be applied in decision-analytic models for individual patients, clinical trials to evaluate new interventions, and population health surveys to compare population groups (Torrance, 1987).

HSUs has the advantage of providing a single cardinal measure of health-related quality of life (HRQoL), suitable for quantitative and parametric statistical analysis (Torrance, 1987). Moreover, it is the only measure that can be used as quality-of-life weights since it captures the strength of individuals' preferences for various health states.

HSUs are cardinal values, reflecting the strength of individuals' preferences for health states, the more preferable a health state, the greater value the state has (Drummond et al., 2005). The cardinal characteristics of

Measuring Health-State Utilities for Cost-Utility Analysis
测量健康效用以用于成本效用分析

HSUs indicate equal intervals on the scale have the same interpretation. For example, health gains from 0.1 to 0.2 and 0.6 to 0.7 on the scale are identical. HSUs should be based on individuals' preferences for health states. It should be noted that the composite scores generated from psychometric or profile-based quality-of-life instruments (e. g. SF-36), which are designed to discriminate different levels of health status, do not necessarily reflect individuals' preferences (Johannesson et al., 1996). It is possible that two individuals have the same level of health but value that health state very differently. HSUs are anchored on full health and death. For convenience, full health and death have been given values of 1.0 and 0, respectively. The advantage of using 1.0 for full health in calculation of QALYs is that the resulting QALYs are measured in the unit of full health year, that is, 1 QALY is one year in full health, 0.5 QALY is half a year in full health, and so on. Health states can also be regarded as worse than death, and take on HSU values less than 0.

When measuring HSUs, three core issues (i. e. how to define health states, how to measure HSUs values, and whose HSUs should be used) need to be addressed (Torrance, 1986; Dolan, 1999; Brazier and Ratcliffe, 2008). In the next sections, these issues will be reviewed. Subsequently, I will provide a description of the research objectives of the project. The last section of the chapter is a brief summary of studies conducted to address the research objectives in this project.

1.1 How to define health states

Health states can be defined through two approaches (Brazier and Ratcliffe, 2008). One is to use bespoke descriptions of health states presented in forms of designed vignettes, text narrative or videos and audios. Another approach is to define health states using standardized health-state classification systems. A health-state classification system consists of a number of multilevel domains. Each health state is defined by combining different levels, one from each domain. Hence, a classification system contains a number of health states. The classification system can be generic, focusing on kernel aspects of health and can be used across all groups, or specific to a certain disease or condition. Taking the classification system of the EQ-5D-3L for example, the system has 5 dimensions (i.e. mobility, self-care, usual activities, pain/discomfort, and anxiety/depression) and each dimension has 3 functional levels (i.e. no problems, some problems, and extreme problems). Together it defines a total of 243 unique health states (i.e. 3^5).

1.2 How to measure HSU values

HSU values can be obtained through valuation techniques such as the standard gamble (SG) (Torrance, 1986) and the time trade-off (TTO) (Torrance, 1972) and preference-based instruments such as the EQ-5D-3L (Dolan, 1997), the health utilities index (HUI) (Feeny et al., 2002), and the short form 6-dimensions (SF-6D) (Brazier et al., 2002). The HSU values can be directly measured from using SG or TTO, whereas the utility value for each health state defined by the classification system of preference-based instruments is pre-determined. In other words, the utility values derived from preference-based instruments are not measured from study subjects. For this reason, the preference-based measures are referred to as indirect methods while the SG and TTO are named as the direct methods.

1.2.1 The direct method

HSUs can be elicited through valuation techniques such as the SG and

TTO. The visual analogue scale (VAS), although also be widely used in health-state valuation, is often criticized due to its scores being elicited in a choiceless context (Green et al., 2000). Moreover, there is empirical evidence of a poor to moderate correlation between VAS values and SG and TTO values (Bakker et al., 1994; Rutten et al., 1995; Clake et al., 1997). Hence, VAS technique seems to measure health status but not the strength of preference for health states (Green et al., 2000). In current health-state valuation practices, VAS is often used as a warm up practice for respondents but not the formal method for eliciting HSUs. Therefore, only SG and TTO are introduced below.

1) Standard gamble

The SG is the classical method for measuring cardinal preferences (Torrance, 1986). It is rooted in the fundamental axioms of expected utility theory (EUT) developed by von Neumann and Morgenstern (1953). The SG has been used extensively in medical decision-making analysis including health-state valuation. The core of the SG is to ask respondents to indicate preferences between a certain intermediate outcome and the uncertainty of a gamble with two possible outcomes: one is better than the certain intermediate outcome while the other is worse.

For health states regarded as better than death (SBTD), the respondent is offered two alternatives (Figure 1.1). Alternative one is a hypothetical treatment with two possible outcomes: either the respondent returns to full health (probability p), or the respondent dies immediately (probability $1-p$). Alternative two is the certain outcome of living in that health state. The probability p is varied until the respondent is indifferent between the two alternatives, at which point the probability p is the utility value for the health state. For health states considered as worse than death (SWTD), the certain alternative is death, whereas the uncertain alternative is living in full health or that health state, with probability p or $1-p$, respectively. Again, the p is varied until the indifference point is reached, at which point the utility value of the health state is $-p/(1-p)$.

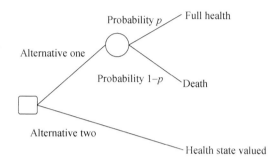

Figure 1.1 SG for a health state considered as better than death

2) Time trade-off

The TTO method was developed specifically for use in health care by Torrance et al(1972). It was designed as a simple-to-administer alternative to SG. Like the SG, it also asks respondents to choose between two alternatives. However, the two alternatives are both under certainty rather than a certain outcome and an uncertain gamble with two outcomes. Essentially, it involves a tradeoff between quantity and quality of life. For SBTD, one alternative is living in a certain period of time (x) in full health and then die; the other alternative is living in a fixed time (t) in the health state valued and then die. Time x is varied until the respondent is indifferent between the two alternatives, at which utility value of the health state is x/t. For SWTD, respondents are also presented with a choice between two alternatives. However, the first alternative is immediate death; the second alternative is time x ($x<t$) in the health state followed by full health until time t and then die. Again, time x is varied until the respondent is indifferent between the two alternatives, at which the utility value for the state is $x-t/x$.

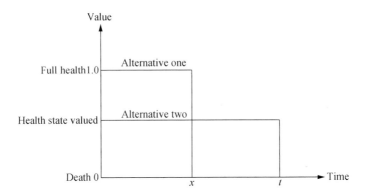

Figure 1.2　TTO for a health state considered as better than death

3) More on standard gamble and time trade-off

The SG is directly rooted in EUT, which has been the dominant theory in decision-making under uncertainty since the 1950s (Dolan, 1999). It postulates a rational individual should make choice between uncertain outcomes in such a way as to obtain the maximum of their "expected" utility or satisfaction. According to the axioms, if a utility is expressed as equivalent to a gamble, it is a linear function of the risk involved in the gamble (Neumann and Morgenstern, 1953). Due to its link with EUT, the SG is often referred to as the "gold standard" for eliciting HSUs (Torrance and Feeny, 1989). However, the status of SG is often criticized by many researchers because of ample evidence for the violation of the axioms of EUT (Froberg and Kane, 1989). For example, the SG values can be significantly influenced by the gamble outcomes in the tasks and the way the tasks presented (Llewellyn-Thomas et al., 1982). Furthermore, there is also evidence suggesting that people's risk attitude is not constant (Kahnerman and Tversky, 1982). Given the empirical violations of the axioms of EUT, the "gold standard" status of the SG for measuring HSUs may not be justifiable.

Compared to the SG, the TTO has the advantage of being simpler to use.

Buckingham and Devlin (2006) aligned the TTO with the welfare economic approach of Compensating Variations (CV) developed by Hicks (1943), where welfare gain is measured by compensating loss of something valuable so that the respondent is returned to their original level of welfare. In the TTO, the health improvement is valued by the corresponding length of life the respondent is prepared to sacrifice. The SG can also be linked with the CV approach, in which the health improvement is valued in terms of the risk (i.e. immediate death) the respondent is prepared to accept. In this way, both the SG and TTO can be viewed as sharing a common theoretical background (Dolan et al., 1996). On the other hand, there are 3 main concerns about the TTO (Green et al., 2000; Brazier and Ratcliffe, 2008). The first is the lack of incorporation of uncertainty. Respondents in the task are asked to make a choice between two certain outcomes, while medical decision in health-care is characterized by its uncertainties. The second is the effect of duration. The TTO assumes that the proportion of remaining life years that individuals are willing to trade off for a specific health improvement is independent of the amount of remaining life. This is a very strong assumption and it seems reasonable to expect that the HSUs may be influenced by the duration effect relating to the time an individual spends in that state (Brazier and Ratcliffe, 2008). The third is the impact of time preference. Individuals may either have positive or negative time preference, meaning they would be either more willing to give up life years in the distant or near future (Drummond et al., 2005).

Both SG and TTO have many variants in terms of mode of administration (e.g. interview or self-administered, computer or paper-based), search procedures (e.g. iteration, titration), the use of prop and visual aids and so on (Torrance, 1987; Dolan et al., 1996; Brazier and Ratcliffe, 2008). Although the two techniques have many types of variants and are cognitive complex, there is empirical evidence to support the practicality of the SG and TTO, with high completion and response rates reported, across different variants and various types of respondent groups (Green et al., 2000; Brazier and Ratcliffe, 2008). Moreover, both techniques demonstrate an acceptable level of test-retest reliability as evidenced by a wide variety of empirical studies (Froberg and Kane, 1989).

Both SG and TTO have important problems in valuing SWTD. First, the valuation procedures for SWTD of the two methods are fundamentally different from their procedures for SBTD. Switching between elicitation procedures for SBTD and SWTD increases the cognitive burden of the tasks for respondents. Second, the denominators are no longer a fixed number in the calculation of negative SG and TTO values, as opposed to the denominators in calculation of positive SG and TTO values. That means the values for SBTD and SWTD may not be measured with the same metric. Third, both techniques can generate extreme negative values and therefore ex post transformation of the negative values to be bounded by -1 is routinely performed in valuation studies using SG or TTO.

To overcome the problems, recently, Robinson and Spencer proposed (2006) and Devlin et al (2011) further developed an approach that unifies the TTO valuation procedures for all health states, which termed as "lead-time TTO (LT-TTO)". The LT-TTO adds a "lead time" in full health preceding each of the two alternatives. The approach avoids the need to have different valuation procedures for SBTD and SWTD by allowing participants to trade the lead time provided. For any health state, the first alternative is x years in full health and then die. The second alternative is z (e.g. 10) years in full health followed by y (e.g. 10) years in the health state and then die. As such, the utility value is $(x-z)/y$. In this case, the utility value will be positive, negative, or 0, depending on the values of $(x-z)$. The approach was found to be a feasible and valid procedure for valuing EQ-5D-3L health states (Devlin et al., 2011) and would be a promising tool in health-state valuation.

Chapter 1
Introduction

4) Discrete choice experiments

The values generated from the SG or TTO may be distorted by factors such as risk aversion (SG), time preference (TTO) and so on (Brazier and Ratcliffe, 2008), indicating the values may not necessarily reflect people's preference over health states. Moreover, both the SG and TTO techniques are cognitively difficult for many respondents, resulting in response inconsistencies and subsequently data exclusions that limit representativeness of the values yielded. Hence, many health services researchers have begun to examine the discrete choice experiments (DCEs), which generate cardinal values from ordinal measurement, in health-state valuation.

The DCEs are based on random utility theory (RUT) proposed by Thurston (1927) and extended by McFadden (1986). Unlike the SG and TTO, respondents in the DCE tasks do not need to go through an iterative process to identify the indifference point between two alternatives. In DCE tasks, each respondent is presented with two or more options and simply required to indicate their most or least preferred options. Through the conditional logistic regression, DCE data can provide estimates on the relative preferences of one option over another. DCE tasks are generally regarded as easier to complete compared to the TTO and SG, and are often conducted without an interviewer through postal or on-line surveys (Brazier and Ratcliffe, 2008).

In health-state valuation, several studies have used DCEs to estimate values for different health-state profiles. However, most of the values are not based on HSU scale, in which 0 is being dead and 1.0 is full health (Bosch JL et al., 1998; Coast et al., 2008). Hence, the DCE data in those studies can not be directly used for calculation of QALYs. Brazier et al(2007) used DCE data to generate health-state values on the health utility scale for the EQ-5D-3L. The use of DCE, although at an early stage of development, offers a promising alternative to the SG and TTO in health-state valuation.

Measuring Health-State Utilities for Cost-Utility Analysis
测量健康效用以用于成本效用分析

1.2.2 The indirect method

The valuation techniques (i.e. TTO and SG) are difficult to administer, cognitively demanding to respondents and resource-intensive to investigators. A widely used alternative is generic preference-based instruments which can be used to obtain HSU values much more easily. The instruments contain two components: a health-state classification system that classifies respondents into various health states using on a questionnaire and a scoring function for scoring these states. The scoring functions are usually established by two steps: first, a subset of possible health states from a classification system are measured using the TTO or SG from a representative sample of a general population; second, these HSU values are used to predict HSU values for all possible health states of the classification system.

There is a wide choice of generic preference-based measures such as the EQ-5D-3L, the HUI marks 2, 3 (HUI2, HUI3), and the SF-6D, a derivative of the SF-36 and SF-12. Among them, the EQ-5D-3L has become most widely used, but others are also be used considerably (Fitzpatrick et al., 2006).

1) EQ-5D-3L

The EQ-5D-3L is a standardized instrument for use as a measure of health outcome developed by the EuroQol Group (Brooks, 1996). The EQ-5D-3L classification system consists of 5 domains: mobility, self-care, usual activities, pain/discomfort, and anxiety/depression, with each domain being described as three levels: "no problems" (level 1); "some problems" (level 2); and "severe problems" (level 3). The system therefore defines a total of 243 (3^5) unique health states. The first scoring algorithm for the EQ-5D-3L health states was derived from the general UK population in the measurement and valuation of health (MVH) study using TTO technique and econometric modeling in 1997 (Dolan, 1997). Subsequently, a number of country-specific

EQ-5D-3L algorithms were developed using a similar research protocol in other countries (Jelsma et al., 2003; Lamers et al., 2006; Shaw et al., 2007; Lee et al., 2009; Golicki et al., 2010).

2) SF-6D

The preference-based instrument SF-6D is a derivative of the SF-36 or SF-12 (an abbreviated version of SF-36 comprising 12 of the SF-36 items) (Brazier et al., 2002; Brazier and Roberts, 2004). The two instruments, although have been widely used in a great number of studies, their scores are not preference-based and therefore can not be used directly in CUA. The SF-6D provides an approach for converting the data collected by SF-36 or SF-12 to HSUs for CUA.

The SF-6D classification system was developed from a selection of 11 SF-36 items (the SF-6D$_{36}$), or 7 SF-12/36 items (the SF-6D$_{12}$). The classification system of the two variants has 6 common domains including physical functioning, role limitations, social functioning, pain, mental health and vitality. The SF-6D$_{36}$ assesses physical functioning, pain, and mental health in greater detail than the SF-6D$_{12}$. Accordingly, the SF-6D$_{12}$ and SF-6D$_{36}$ define 7,500 and 18,000 unique health states, respectively. The scoring algorithms for SF-6D$_{36}$ and SF-6D$_{12}$ were constructed using the same random sample of the general UK population based on SG technique and econometric modeling method.

3) HUI

The HUI is a family of generic preference-based system for measuring comprehensive health status and HRQoL (Feeny et al., 1995; Torrance et al., 1995). There are currently two HUI systems: HUI2 and HUI3. The classification system of HUI2 consists of 6 domains (i.e. sensation, mobility, emotion, cognition, self-care, and pain), each with 4 to 5 levels. The HUI3 classification system has 8 domains: vision, hearing, speech,

Measuring Health-State Utilities for Cost-Utility Analysis
测量健康效用以用于成本效用分析

ambulation, dexterity, emotion, cognition, and pain, with 3 to 5 levels per domain. The two systems define a total of 24,000, and 972,000 health states, respectively. The scoring functions for the two systems were based on SG values derived from random samples of the general Canadian population and estimated using a multiplicative model.

Although these measures all claim to measure generic health (i.e. important aspects of health appropriate for all populations), they do differ significantly in terms of the content and capacity of their classification system, valuation technique, source of population used to value health states, and scoring methods. A summary of the main characteristics of these measures is presented in Table 1.1.

Table 1.1 Characteristics of the generic preference-based instruments

	EQ-5D-3L	SF-6D$_{36}$	SF-6D$_{12}$	HUI2	HUI3
Classification system					
Dimension or attribute (number of levels)	Mobility(3)	PF(6)	PF(3)	Mobility(5)	Ambulation(6)
	AD(3)	MH(5)	MH(5)	Emotion(5)	Emotion(5)
	PD(3)	BP(6)	BP(5)	Pain(5)	Pain(5)
	UA(3)	SF(5)	SF(5)	Cognition(4)	Cognition(6)
	Self-care(3)	RL(4)	RL(4)	Self-care(4)	Dexterity(6)
		Vitality(5)	Vitality(5)	Sensation(4)	Hearing(6)
					Speech(5)
					Vision(6)
Number of health states defined	243	18,000	7,500	24,000	972,000
Utility score					
Valuation technique	TTO	SG	SG	SG	SG
Country and Region where the utilities are from	US, UK, Japan, Denmark, Zimbabwe etc	UK, HK, Japan, Brazil, etc	UK	Canada, UK	Canada, France

(To be continued)

Chapter 1
Introduction

(Continued)

	EQ-5D-3L	SF-6D$_{36}$	SF-6D$_{12}$	HUI2	HUI3
Scoring method	Statistical-additive model with interaction	Statistical-additive model with interaction	Statistical-additive model with interaction	MAUT-multiplicative function	MAUT-multiplicative function

PF: physical functioning; MH: mental health; BP: bodily pain; SF: social functioning; RL: role limitations; AD: anxiety/depression; PD: pain/discomfort; UA: usual activities. MAUT: multi-attribute utility theory

Given the differences mentioned above, it is not surprising that these measures have produced different utility values for the same respondents (McDonough and Tosteson, 2007). Then the question is how to select an appropriate instrument.

In selecting an instrument, researchers should consider a number of factors including feasibility, psychometric properties (i.e. validity, reliability, sensitivity and responsiveness), the degree of the overlap between the levels and dimensions of the classification system and the target population, respondent burden, overall cost of using the instrument and so on (Drummond et al., 2005).

One issue regarding the instrument selection is the generalizability of HSU values from the instruments. Since the HSU values are initially scored based on one particular population, these values may not reflect people's value of health in other populations. Although some researchers replicated HSUs measurements (i.e. controlling for method) in different populations and found either no or little difference (Drummond et al., 2005), some other investigators showed that HSUs differed significantly across different populations in different countries (Norman et al., 2009). Hence, recent years have seen an increasing number of studies developing country-specific HSU value sets (Jelsma et al., 2003; Lamers et al., 2006; Shaw et al., 2007; Lee et al., 2009; Golicki et al., 2010)

A general limitation of generic preference-based instruments is that they may lack sensitivity and relevance to particular diseases or conditions. As a result, the disease-specific preference-based measures have started to emerge in the literature (Revicki et al., 1998; Yang et al., 2006; Brazier et al., 2008). However, it is questionable that whether the utility values from these measures are generalizable or comparable across different patient groups. These are important in economic evaluations in which the purpose is to inform resource allocation decisions across different patient groups. Ultimately, for both generic and disease-specific preference-based measures, there is a trade-off between the greater relevance and sensitivity of some and limited generalizability.

1.2.3 Mapping health profiles to health-state utilities

HSU data collected by preference-based instruments may not always be available. In such situations, mapping, that is the development and use of a function (or functions) to predict HSU values using data on non-preference-based measure or profile-based measure, can be the solution (NICE, 2013). The data for predicting HSU values can be the condition-specific instruments (e.g. Parkinson's Disease Questionnaire), generic instruments (e.g. SF-36), clinical indicators of disease severity, socio-demographic variables or a combination of these.

The approach involves using regression model to estimate the relationship between preference-based measure and profile-based measure and requires administration of the two measures to the same population, and sufficient similarity in item content between the two measures. Once the mapping function established, it can be applied to data collected using the profile-based measure to predict HSU values.

Recent years have seen an increasing number of studies developing functions to predict preference scores from psychometric quality-of-life instruments. Such approach has been accepted as a valid method for yielding utility scores by National Institute for Health and Care Excellence

(NICE)(2012).

1) Model specification

Mapping functions can be established using a number of specifications and different estimation methods. The most widely used model is additive model: the dependent variables can be the index scores of target preference-based instruments or dimension levels of the instruments; the independent variables can be the overall scores, dimension scores, item scores, or item responses to profile-based measure (Brazier et al., 2010). Among them, overall scores, dimension scores and item scores are treated as continuous variables but item responses are modeled as categorical variables and dummy variables are generated for each item response. To relax the assumptions of simple additive model, the square and interaction terms for dimension or item scores can also be included as independent variables. In addition, non-health variables such as age, gender and race can also be used as independent variables.

2) Model estimation

The most common method of estimating mapping functions has been the ordinary least square (OLS) model (Brazier et al., 2010). However, the classical OLS assumptions are deviated and violated in many dataset which will generally cause the estimates to be biased, inconsistent and/or inefficient. For example, if the utility scores exhibit a ceiling effect, that is, a large proportion of respondents have a utility score of 1.0, the OLS model may lead to predicted values outside the theoretical range of the utility scale. Hence, researchers have explored alternatives of OLS model to overcome its limitations, including Tobit model, censored least absolute deviation (CLAD) model, latent-class model and two-part models which are appropriate for censored or bounded data. For such data, these models were compared with OLS but the results were mixed with some indicating the

CLAD and two-part models performed better than the OLS model (Sullivan and Ghushchyan, 2006), others concluding that the CLAD and OLS models had similar performance (Eleanor et al., 2010).

3) Model performance

Model performance can be assessed by a number of criteria such as consistency, bias, and precision. Consistency means the model should predict lower utility scores for more severe health problems. Precision is the accuracy of the predictions, which can be evaluated using a number of goodness-of-fit measures such as adjusted R^2, mean error (ME), mean absolute error (MAE) and root mean squared error (RMSE). Adjusted R^2 tells how well the model explains the variance of actual values in the estimation dataset, and the other measures examine the average difference between predicted and observed values and provide a quantitative view of the prediction errors. In addition, numbers or proportion of absolute errors greater or smaller than some thresholds (e.g. 0.05 or 5%) can also be used to compare models' performance. Prediction errors can be assessed at individual-level or aggregate-level. Bias refers to the pattern of prediction errors across the scale of the dependent variable. If there are systematic errors in the predictions, researchers need to consider the impact of the bias on the CUA.

A recent review of mapping studies suggested that mapping from condition-specific quality-of-life measure onto a generic preference-based measure has poorer model performance than mapping from generic quality-of-life measure onto a generic preference-based measure (Brazier et al., 2010). This is due to limited degree of overlap in item content between the preference-based measure and condition-specific measure as important dimensions of one measure may not be covered by the other. An alternative in these situations is to derive disease-specific preference-based measures.

Ideally, model performance should be both assessed on the estimation dataset which is used to construct the model and on an external dataset similar to the estimation dataset. Nevertheless, it is not uncommon that the external dataset is unavailable. In that case, if the original dataset is large in size, it is recommended to randomly split the data into an "estimation" sample and a "validation" sample. The model is estimated on the "estimation" sample and its performance is checked using the "validation" sample. Once the model specification has been evaluated and determined, the final model can then be re-estimated using the full sample.

The main advantage of mapping is that it enables HSU values to be predicted when only health profile data is available. However, as the mapping functions just predict rather than measure HSU values directly, which will lead to increased uncertainty and error for the estimated HSU values, using mapping functions is always a second best solution to using preference-based instruments.

1.3 Whose health-state utilities should be used

HSUs can be elicited from different sources such as patient and general populations (Torrance, 1986). For the purpose of personal clinical decisions, it is clear that patient utilities should be used. On the other hand, for decisions about allocating societal resources, there is the question of whose utilities should be used and the question has been intensively debated in the literature (Boyd et al., 1990; Ulber et al., 2001; Brazier et al., 2005; Chapman et al., 2009). The question is of great importance as it may influence the resultant utility values. According to a meta-analysis, on average, there is no significant difference in HSUs between patient and general populations (Dolders et al., 2006); however, for some disease, differences do exist. A number of empirical studies have indicated that patients who are experiencing certain diseases tend to give higher health-state utilities than members of the general population (Sackett and Torrance,

1978; Llewellyn-Thomas et al., 1982; Boyd et al., 1990; Hurst et al., 1994), and the extent of this discrepancy tends to be much stronger when patients value their own health state (Brazier et al., 2005).

The difference described above can have important consequences in CUA in health care. For example, if patients with colostomies rate their own HSU as 0.92 while those without colostomies estimate the utility of living with a colostomy as 0.80, and the magnitude of incremental gain from a treatment avoids the need for a colostomy and restores patients to full health (1.0) would be more than twice using utility value from the non-patients than patients with colostomies.

The difference could be attributed to various factors such as poor descriptions of health states to general population (Ulber et al., 2003), response shift (i.e. changes in internal standards of health) or adaptation (Ulber et al., 2003), and cognitive dissonance (Festinger L, 1957).

1.3.1 General population health-state utilities

HSUs are normally obtained from members of the general population trying to imagine and value health states of patients. The main argument for the use of general population utility values is that societal resource allocation decisions should be made appealing to the whole society since the general population pays for healthcare services. Relatedly, if one of the purposes of the healthcare system is to give reassurance to the general public, resources should, in part, be allocated so as to reassure the public that treatment is available to alleviate the health problems they fear the most (Edgar et al., 1998). On the other hand, although members of the general public want to be involved in healthcare decision making, it is not clear whether HSUs or QALYs are their main considerations. Furthermore, members of the general population in the current valuation practice are relatively uninformed: they are unlikely to know about the consequences of disease and other changes.

Hence, their values will not reflect what it is actually like to be in the health state. Nevertheless, the Washington Panel used the "veil of ignorance" to support the use of community values, where a rational public decides what is the best course of action when blind to its own self-interest. Aggregating the utilities of persons who have no vested interest in particular health states seems most appropriate (Gold et al., 1996).

1.3.2 Patient health-state utilities

The argument for using patient values is that patients know their health states and the impact of their health problems better than those trying to imagine them. However, this would imply that society wants to incorporate all the changes and adaptations that occur in patients who experience states of ill health. Furthermore, there is evidence suggesting that patient values are not constant, and reflecting their recent experiences of ill health or the health of their relatives or close friends (Kind and Dolan, 1995). In addition, valuation techniques (i.e. SG, TTO) require respondents to compare their own state to full health, which patients may not have experienced for a long time. The tasks of imagining full health can be as difficult for patients as members of the general public imagining dysfunctional health states.

In summary, it is difficult to justify the exclusive use of utility values from patients or members of the general public. The question of whose utility values should be used is a normative judgment. If it is accepted that, ultimately, the utility values of general population are required to inform resource allocation in a public system, the respondents should be provided with adequate information on what the states are like for patients experiencing them (Brazier et al., 2005). Meanwhile, empirical studies are needed to compare HSU values between patient and general population for various diseases.

Measuring Health-State Utilities for Cost-Utility Analysis
测量健康效用以用于成本效用分析

1.4 Research objectives

The overall object of the book was to develop and test various approaches to measuring health-state utilities for cost-utility analysis.

The increasing application of CUA to evaluate cost-effectiveness of health interventions has led to an increased demand for HSUs for usage in various populations and settings. In Singapore, we recognized that there was no local HSU value sets and studies often use off-the-shelf HSU value sets developed from other populations (Luo et al., 2003a; Luo et al., 2003b; Luo et al., 2003c; Luo et al., 2009; Gao et al., 2009; Abdin et al., 2009; Zhang et al., 2009; Wang et al., 2012; Chong et al., 2012). However, it is unlikely that HSU values are universal, although some studies do indicate the similarities of HSUs across countries (Wang et al., 2002; Le Gale et al., 2002). Hence, the first objective of this project was to compare the HSU values of Singaporeans and the people in China, and the second objective was to establish an EQ-5D-3L value set using time trade-off (TTO) values directly measured from the general Singaporean population.

The impact of using different sources (i.e. patient and general population) of HSUs is important, as for some diseases, the difference in HSU values do exist and may have significant impact on the CUA of health interventions (Sackett and Torrance, 1978; Llewellyn-Thomas et al., 1982; Boyd et al., 1990; Hurst et al., 1994). Whether the divergence in patients and general population HSU values exists and what's the impact of the divergence need to be assessed for different clinical conditions. Thus, the third objective of this project was to compare the utility values for EQ-5D-3L health states between type 2 diabetes mellitus (T2DM) patients and the general population in Singapore.

Although research on generating HSU values has grown considerably, there is still a lack of valid approaches in many situations. For example, the data collected by psychometric instruments which are designed to reflect individuals' health status but not their preferences for health states can not be directly used to calculate QALYs. In such situations, HSU values need to be obtained through the use of mapping that converts the non-preference-based data into preference scores (Brazier et al., 2010). Hence, the fourth objective of this project was to develop and test functions for predicting the preference-based SF-6D$_{36}$ index scores from the SF-8 health survey (Ware et al., 2001).

Selecting the most appropriate preference-based instrument is important as different instruments appear to yield different HSU values for the same health profiles. Generic preference-based instruments such as EQ-5D-3L (Dolan, 1997), SF-6D$_{12}$ (Brazier and Roberts, 2004), SF-6D$_{36}$ (Brazier et al., 2002), and HUI2 and HUI3 (Feeny et al., 1995; Torrance et al., 1995) differ significantly in various aspects. Thus, the fifth objective of this project was to compare the discriminative power of the SF-6D index scores derived from the SF-36 (SF-6D$_{36}$) and SF-12 (SF-6D$_{12}$) in the general population.

1.5 Summary of studies

The subsequent five chapters are devoted to studies used to address the above five research objectives, with each chapter for one study.

The 2nd chapter reports a study of comparing the preference values for EQ-5D-5L health states between Chinese Singaporean and the people in China. In this study, the preference values for 10 selected EQ-5D-5L health states were elicited using TTO method from a convenience sample of Singaporeans and a convenience sample of Chinese in Beijing. The difference in TTO values between Mainland Chinese in Singapore and three subgroups of Singaporeans (i.e. English-speaking Chinese [EC], Chinese-speaking Chinese

[CC], and non-Chinese [NC]) was analyzed using random-effects linear regression and logistic regression models.

The 3rd chapter reports a study of exploring the impact of diabetes on HSUs, using data collected from a consecutive sample of outpatients with T2DM in the National University Hospital (NUH). T2DM patients' utility values for EQ-5D-3L health states were compared with values from a general Singapore population sample also using random-effects linear regression and logistic regression models.

The 4th chapter reports a valuation study of establishing the Singapore EQ-5D-3L value set. In this study, the values of 80 EQ-5D-3L health states were directly elicited from a general Singaporean population sample using a TTO method. Various linear regression models and model specifications were examined to assess their goodness of fit to the data, at both aggregate and individual levels, and ability to predict the values for unmeasured EQ-5D-3L health states.

The 5th chapter reports a mapping study of developing a function for yielding the preference-based $SF-6D_{36}$ index score from the $SF-8$ health survey, using data collected in a population health survey in which respondents ($n = 7,529$) completed both the SF-36 and the SF-8 questionnaires. Various OLS models were assessed for their performance in predicting the $SF-6D_{36}$ score from the SF-8 at both the individual and the group level.

The 6th chapter reports a study comparing the discriminative power of the SF-6D index score derived from the SF-36 ($SF-6D_{36}$) and SF-12 ($SF-6D_{12}$) in the general population, using data from a sample of the general US adult population. The discriminative power of the $SF-6D_{36}$ and $SF-6D_{12}$ were compared using F-statistic and Shannon index (H').

Chapter 2

Do Chinese Have Similar Health-State Preferences? A Comparison of the People in China and Chinese Singaporeans

2.1 Introduction

Given the relatively rare resources and rapidly rising costs of health services and technologies, cost-utility analysis (CUA) comparing the costs of a service or technology with its benefits from the societal perspective is increasingly used for setting priorities (Bloom, 2004). In CUA, the benefits are measured in terms of quality-adjusted life-years (QALYs) that combines both the quality and quantity of life. In order to obtain the quality-of-life weights for calculating QALYs, researchers need to measure the general public's preferences for the relevant health outcomes (Gold et al., 1996). The preference values of health outcomes are measured on an interval scale on which 1 is full health, 0 is death, and negative values correspond to health states regarded as worse than death (Drummond et al., 2005).

Preference-based instruments such as the EQ-5D-3L (Dolan, 1997), the health utilities index (HUI) (Feeny et al., 2002) and the short form 6-dimensions ($SF-6D_{36}$) (Brazier, 2002) are designed to measure the value of health services or technologies to the society. Such instruments comprise a questionnaire for describing individuals' health and a set of values indicating the value of the health states it describes to the general public. The values are estimated based on empirically measured health-state preferences from a general population sample using valuation techniques such as the time trade-off (TTO) (Torranc et al., 1972) and standard gamble (SG) (Torrance, 1986).

Whether the general populations in different countries have different health-state preferences is an important issue in economic evaluation of health services and technologies. If the preferences of different populations are systematically different and could lead to different CUA results, it is necessary to use local preference value sets in CUA; otherwise, the preferences estimated from one particular population could be applied to other populations, and the resources and time spent for developing local preference value sets can be saved.

To date, a number of studies compared health-state preferences across different populations (Drummond et al., 2005; Badia et al., 2001; Luo et al., 2007; Wang et al., 2002; Norman et al., 2009; Tsuchiya et al., 2002; Johnson et al., 2005). However, the findings are mixed. Some studies suggested that the differences in health-state preferences across populations are either absent or negligible (Drummond et al., 2005). Other studies indicated that health-state preferences differ significantly among different populations and may influence the results of CUA. For example, a recent review of the TTO values for EQ-5D-3L health states found that compared to the range of UK TTO values, the ranges of Japan and US TTO values are narrower, which could lead to less cost-effectiveness in CUA (Norman et al., 2009). It should be noted that many of those studies have the limitation of using pooled data from independent studies in which different valuation procedures were used. It has been well demonstrated that different variants of the prevailing valuation methods such as SG and TTO lead to systematically different health-state values (Dolan et al., 1996).

We are particularly interested in the issue of whether Chinese in different regions have similar health-state preferences given the fact that Chinese mainly live in several geographically distinct areas (e.g. the mainland

Chapter 2
Do Chinese Have Similar Health-State Preferences? A Comparison of the People in China and Chinese Singaporeans

of China, the Hongkong of China, the Taiwan of China, the Macau of China and Singapore) and there is no study comparing the preference values among Chinese populations in different regions. For this purpose, we conducted a head-to-head comparison of the TTO preference values for EQ-5D-5L health states elicited from the people in China and Chinese Singaporeans who form 74.2% of the Singaporean population (Department of Statistic Singapore, 2013) using data from a multi-national study.

2.2 Methods

The data used in this study was from the multinational pilot valuation study of the EQ-5D-5L health states (Oppe et al., 2012). This valuation study collected data from 8 general population samples, each from a different country. Investigators in each study site collected data using a standard procedure to answer a common primary research question, although they also collected additional data using slightly different procedures to address various secondary research questions. Since the current study only used data from the mainland of China and Singapore, study designs used in the two countries were described below.

2.2.1 Sampling and recruitment

The study samples in the mainland of China and Singapore were drawn in a similar way. In both sites, the sampling frame was on a large cohort of general population members maintained by a commercial research company. Members from the Singapore cohort were from all over Singapore and had good computer skills since they participated in on-line surveys periodically; members of the Chinese cohort mainly resided in Beijing, the capital of China where many residents were immigrated from other regions of China.

In both study sites, members in the sampling frames were randomly selected and personally invited through telephone by the research companies. Stratified random sampling was conducted in the recruitment process in order to achieve samples with balanced distributions of gender and age groups. Participants' eligibility was checked twice during the recruitment and on the day of survey using the following criteria: 1) aged 18 years or above; 2) literate and able to read text from a computer screen; 3) able to use a mouse and Internet Explorer to surf the Internet; 4) able to give informed consent. Literacy was defined as able to read English or Chinese newspapers and to converse fluently in either language.

2.2.2 Procedures

Consenting participants were invited in small groups to a computer room to complete a survey in the manner of computer-assisted self interviewing (CASI). Each participant was assigned to a computer on which the EQ-VT program was run to administer the survey questions. Participants were asked to independently complete the survey after a group demonstration of how the interview software program works. Investigators were around the room to provide assistance if any participant encountered any difficulties. Participants received a monetary incentive worth approximately 15 Euros on completion of the survey. In accordance to a standard study protocol, the target sample size was 400 in both study sites.

2.2.3 EQ-VT

The EQ-VT is a software package developed by the EuroQol Group (www.euroqol.org) for collecting raw valuation data of the EQ-5D-5L health states. It was designed for use in the mode of CASI. The Chinese version of EQ-VT was translated by a professional translation company from

English into Chinese and tested extensively for technical issues and understandability in the target populations.

The survey was programmed into four sections. The questions in the first section were for warm-up purpose. Participants in the section were asked to rate their own health status using the EQ-5D-5L questionnaire and provide background information on their age and gender. The EQ-5D-5L questionnaire contains two parts: the EQ-5D-5L classification system and the EQ visual analogue scale (EQ-VAS). The classification system is a new version of the EQ-5D-3L, which has the same 5 domains as the EQ-5D-3L, but is with 5 descriptive levels (EuroQol Group, 2013). The EQ-VAS can record participants' own health on a vertical visual analogue. The second section collected valuation data for 10 selected pairs of different EQ-5D-5L health states. The third section included 5 TTO tasks for measuring preference values of 5 EQ-5D-5L health states. The questions in the last section collected participants' feedback and comments on the survey questions.

The TTO tasks in the third section were presented using either standard or experimental arms. In both sites, participants were randomized to one arm and one block of health states ($n = 5$). The TTO tasks in the standard arm were the same for the two sites but have some differences in the experimental arm which was reported elsewhere (Luo et al., 2013). Only the data collected from the standard arm was used in the current study.

In the standard arm, each state was valued using a series of questions each asking the participant's preference between two hypothetical lives: living in full health for 10 years followed by 5 years in the state valued and then die (Life A) and living x years ($0 \leqslant x \leqslant 15$) in full health and then die (Life B). For each question, the participant's response could be Life A, Life B, or A & B are about the same. If the response was life A or Life B, a new question with a different x value would be presented to the participant. The questioning would stop when the response was "A & B are about the same". In this case, the current valuation task would end and a new task for a different health state would start. How the x values changed was reported elsewhere (Oppe et al., 2012). Briefly, the first two values of x were 15 and 10 years. The third value for x was 12.5 (or 5) years if the answer to the second question was Life A (or Life B). The x values in subsequent questions varied with a unit from 3 months to 1 year depending on participants' responses.

Since limited numbers of x values were programmed in the EQ-VT, some participants may not answer "A & B are about the same" for some health states at any provided x values. In such cases, the available x value closest to the indifference point between the two lives would be used as the indifference point.

2.2.4 Health states valued

The health states valued in the study were defined by the EQ-5D-5L health-state classification system. The classification system comprises 5 domains (i.e. mobility, self-care, usual activities, pain/discomfort, and anxiety/depression), and each domain has 5 functional levels including no problem (level 1), slight problems (level 2), moderate problems (level 3), severe problems (level 4), and extreme problems (level 5). Each EQ-5D-5L state can be expressed by a 5-digit number. For example, 12345 represents no problem in mobility, slight problems in self-care, moderate problems in usual activities, severe problems in pain or discomfort, and extreme problems in anxiety or depression. The 10 EQ-5D-5L states selected by the EQ-VT spread over various severities, including 12112, 52221, 33133, 44113 and 53555 in one block, 21111, 11221, 52324, 55523 and 11145 in the other block. The EQ-5D-5L health states were divided into two categories: states with and without severe health problems. Two or three states were randomly selected from each category to construct a block of 5 states.

2.2.5 Data analysis

Participants were excluded if they valued all states the same, which was regarded as not really understand the valuation tasks; non-Chinese participants from Singapore were also excluded. In addition, TTO values were excluded if they only spend 1 second on the task, which was considered as unreliable. The characteristics of the people in China and Chinese Singaporean participants were compared using Chi-square tests or Fisher's exact tests for categorical variables and two-sample t-tests for continuous variables.

The TTO value for each EQ-5D-5L health state valued was calculated as $U = (T - 10)/5$, in which U is the TTO value and $T (0 \leqslant T \leqslant 15 \text{ years})$ is the time at which indifference was reached. The possible range of the TTO values was therefore from -2 ($T = 0$) to 1 ($T = 15$).

Data collected from the two populations were pooled for a series of regression analysis. First, the TTO values for all the 10 health states were analyzed using a linear regression model. Second, the TTO values for states with mild or moderate problems (i.e. 11221, 12112, 21111 and 33133), states with severe or extreme problems (i.e. 44113, 11145, 52324, 53555 and 55523) and each of the 10 health states were investigated using separate linear regression models. Third, whether the people in China and Chinese Singaporeans have different tendency to rate the health states as worse than death (i.e. TTO values <0) was investigated using logistic regression model. In all models, the TTO value was regressed on the source of the value (Chinese Singaporeans or the people in China) with and without the adjustment of other factors. The factors adjusted for included age, gender, TTO block, and self-reported health problems in EQ-5D-5L domains. All adjusted factors were coded into dummy variables. For the health-state characteristics, five dummy variables were generated to specify the existence of any health problems in each of the domains of a health state. The random effects were built into the models to adjust for individual cluster of data in which participants gave multiple TTO values.

2.3 Results

A total of 210 participants completed the valuation survey using standard visual aids in the mainland of China study. After excluding 16 participants who gave same TTO values for all the 5 health states and 6 valuation tasks that were completed within 1 second, 964 TTO values derived from 194 participants were used in this analysis. The mean age of the participants was 36.5 years old, with male being 50.0%. The majority of them did not experience any problems in EQ-5D health domains on the day of the survey (58.2%) (Table 2.1).

In the Singapore study, 2 Chinese Singaporean participants were excluded since they valued all health states same and 50 non-Chinese participants were excluded. After that, 145 participants with 725 observations of TTO values were included in the analysis. The mean age of the participants was 37.6 years old, with male being 53.1%. The majority of them was English-speaking (62.8%), and many of them did not experience any problems in EQ-5D health domains on the day of the survey (48.7%) (Table 2.1).

Table 2.1 Characteristics of participants

	N(%)		P value
	the people in China $N = 194$	Chinese Singaporeans $N = 145$	
Gender			0.3525
Male	97(50.0)	77(53.1)	
Female	97(50.0)	68(46.9)	
Age group, year			0.4663
18-44 years	144(74.2)	108(71.7)	
>44 years	50(25.8)	41(28.3)	

(To be continued)

Chapter 2
Do Chinese Have Similar Health-State Preferences? A Comparison of the People in China and Chinese Singaporeans

(Continued)

	N(%)		P value
	the people in China N = 194	Chinese Singaporeans N = 145	
Interview language			<0.0001
Chinese	194(100)	54(37.2)	
English	0(0)	91(62.8)	
Mobility			0.0015
No problems	191(98.4)	139(95.9)	
With problems	3(1.6)	6(4.1)	
Self-care			0.1958
No problems	192(99.0)	142(97.9)	
With problems	2(1.0)	3(2.1)	
Usual activity			0.0919
No problems	189(97.4)	138(95.2)	
With problems	5(2.6)	7(4.8)	
Pain/discomfort			<0.0001
No problems	143(73.7)	86(59.3)	
With problems	51(26.3)	59(40.7)	
Anxiety/depression			0.3689
No problems	138(71.1)	108(74.5)	
With problems	56(28.9)	37(25.5)	
VAS, mean (SD)	89.5(9.1)	84.6(10.1)	<0.0001
TTO block			0.2129
1	97(50.0)	65(44.8)	
2	97(50.0)	80(55.2)	

Chi-square tests or Fisher's exacts test for categorical variables and two sample t-tests for continuous variables; SD: standard deviation

Participants from the two populations differed significantly in some aspects. For example, the participants of China reported better overall health, and were less likely to experience health problems in EQ-5D domains (Table 2.1).

All 10 EQ-5D-5L health states considered, the mean TTO value was 0.18 for Chinese Singaporeans and 0.35 for the people in China, with the difference(95% confidence interval [95% CI]) being 0.17(0.07, 0.28); the proportion of TTO values < 0 for Chinese Singaporeans (21.2%) was higher than that for the people in China(18.8%), with the odds ratio(95% CI) of giving a negative value for Singapore versus the mainland of China being

1.41(0.89, 2.24). The mean TTO values of the people in China and Chinese Singaporeans were similar when the values for states with mild or moderate problems were considered; while the people in China had substantially higher TTO values for states with severe or extreme health problems (Table 2.2). The mean difference(95%CI) between the two populations was 0.04(−0.07, 0.15) for the former, and 0.32(0.19, 0.44) for the latter. The magnitude of these differences remained similar after adjusting for other variables (Table 2.2).

Table 2.2 Comparison of TTO values between the people in China and Chinese Singaporeans

	the people in China	Chinese Singaporeans	Difference between the people in China and Chinese Singaporeans*	
	Mean (SD)	Mean (SD)	Unadjusted(95%CI)	Adjusted(95%CI)†
All health states	0.35(0.60)	0.18(0.75)	−0.17(−0.28, −0.07)	−0.16(−0.27, −0.05)
Health states with mild or moderate problems	0.45(0.55)	0.49(0.61)	0.04(−0.07, 0.15)	0.04(−0.07, 0.15)
Health states with severe or extreme problems	0.28(0.61)	−0.04(0.76)	−0.32(−0.44, −0.19)	−0.30(−0.42, −0.17)
TTO values<0, N (%)	181(18.8)	123(21.2)	OR(95%CI) 1.41(0.89, 2.24)	OR(95%CI) 1.39(0.86, 2.24)‡

CI: confidence interval; SD: standard deviation; OR: odds ratio

* Reference group is the people in China and the random effect was used in the comparison analyses with and without adjustment

† Random effect linear regression model, in which age group, gender, TTO block, and self-reported health problems in EQ-5D-5L health domains

‡ Random effect logistic regression model, in which age group, gender, TTO block, and self-reported health problems in EQ-5D-5L health domains

The mean values of individual health states varied from −0.21 (for 53555) to 0.57 (for 12112) for Chinese Singaporeans and from 0.19 (for 53555) to 0.50 (for 21111) for the people in China (Figure 2.1), with the range being 0.78 and 0.31 for Chinese Singaporeans and the people in China, respectively. Difference in the mean TTO values was less than 0.10 for four states in which only slightly or moderate problems are present in one or more of the EQ-5D health dimensions (i.e. 11221, 12112, 21111, and 33133). On the other hand, the difference ranged from 0.19 to 0.40 for the remaining six states in which at least one health dimension is described as having severe or extreme problems, with statistical significance observed in four of the states where the largest differences occurred (Figure 2.1).

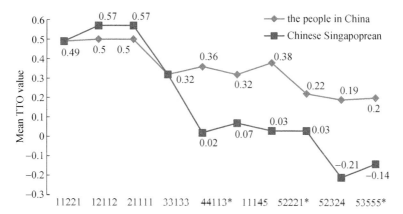

Figure 2.1 Mean TTO values for each of the 10 EQ-5D-5L health states between the people in China and Chinese Singaporeans

* Difference in TTO values between the people in China and Chinese Singaporeans is statistically significant with adjustment of age, gender, TTO block, and self-reported health problems in EQ-5D-5L health domains

2.4 Discussion

To the best our knowledge, this was the first study comparing directly measured health-state preference values between two Chinese populations. Previous studies compared between different western populations (Badia et al., 2001; Johnson et al., 2005; Johnson et al., 2000) or between an Asian population and a western population (Tsuchiya et al., 2002). Moreover, those studies used data collected from independent studies conducted in different times by different investigators. In contrast, data used in our study was collected by the same investigators using exactly the same study protocol, thus ruling out the effects of some unobservable confounders in the comparison. Hence, our study provides important information on the similarity or difference in health-state preferences among Chinese populations because it has shown differences in health state valuation in two Chinese populations using exactly the same study design and protocol.

We found that Chinese Singaporeans valued EQ-5D-5L health states lower, that they were more likely to rate a health state as worse than death, and more importantly, that they valued states with severe or extreme problems as much more undesirable than the people in China. This result suggests that the health benefit gained from a transition from a severe health state to a mild health is much greater to Chinese Singaporeans than to the people in China. For example, according to our study, the gain from transition between 11145 and 12112 would be 0.43 and 0.18 to Chinese Singaporeans and the people in China, respectively. This means a health service or technology which can achieve such an improvement in health would be considered much more cost-effective to Chinese Singaporeans than the people in China, if the associated costs are similar. Therefore, an important implication of our study is that a local value set for EQ-5D-5L health states should be used in cost-utility analysis to Chinese Singaporeans since using the EQ-5D-5L values of the people in China could underestimate the value of health technologies of investigation. Hence, our study supports the development of local EQ-5D-5L preference value sets in these two Chinese regions to inform decision making for health resource allocation.

The difference in TTO values between the two countries should be due to the fact that poor life is more undesirable than short life to Chinese Singaporeans compared to the people in China. This may be attributed to two reasons: medical costs and attitude towards death and longevity. First, medical costs are mainly borne by individuals and their immediate family members in Singapore. As a result, Singaporeans including Chinese Singaporeans may be more willing to give up life years in order to reduce financial burden due to poor health. A recent study in Singapore found that cancer patients would not choose to use better but more expensive treatment if they had to pay for the treatment (BMJ Group Blogs, 2013). In contrast,

Chapter 2
Do Chinese Have Similar Health-State Preferences? A Comparison of the People in China and Chinese Singaporeans

the majority of health expenses can be reimbursed for urban residents (e.g. residents in Beijing) in the mainland of China (World Health Organization, 2013). It should be noted that respondents to TTO or other health-state valuation questions should not consider the economic consequences of the health problems to be valued. However, it would be difficult for respondents to follow exactly such instructions if in reality health services are not free. Second, most people in China prefer to have a longer life. In a recent study, 50.3% of the people in China endorsed that: "a living dog is better than a dead lion" and that 72.8% of participants reported that they do not believe life after death. Singaporeans might be less afraid of death because 83% of the population believed in certain religion (Singapore Department of Statistics, 2013) as compared to about 20% in the mainland of China (BBC News, 2013). Nevertheless, those reasons are speculative, future studies should further explore the impact of death and longevity attitudes on health-state valuations.

There were two limitations in this study. First, in both countries, the stratified random sampling method was used and all participants recruited possessed some levels of computer skills. Moreover, the participants of China were mainly from Beijing. Hence, the generalizability of our findings may be limited. Second, the TTO valuation tasks were self-administered although assistance would be provided on participants' request. As a result, some participants might not fully understand the tasks and gave erroneous responses (Oppe et al., 2012), which may reduce the statistical power and even the validity of our findings. Due to these limitations, the finding of our study should be treated with caution.

In conclusion, the TTO values of EQ-5D-5L health states differ between the people of China and Chinese Singaporeans, which could lead to different CUA results if one population's preferences are used to the other population. Hence, local EQ-5D-5L value sets should be developed wherever possible.

Chapter 3

The Impact of Diabetes on Health-State Utilities

3.1 Introduction

Utility of health technologies is usually evaluated using health-state utilities elicited from general or patient populations. While there seems to be a consensus that patients should be the source of utility values in the context of clinical decision making (Gold et al., 1996; Dobrez et al., 2007; Revicki et al., 2011), whose values should be used in analysis intended to inform allocation of societal health resources has long been debated (Dolan, 1999(a); Dolan, 1999(b); Ulber et al., 2003; Ulber et al., 2000; Brazier et al., 2005; Gandjour, 2010). The main argument for using the values elicited from the general population is that members of the general population are the payers and potential users of health technologies and services. On the other hand, Gandjour argued that only patient utilities have a theoretical foundation in preference-utilitarian theory and welfare economics (2010). The issue of whose values to use is based on the assumption that the health-state preferences of the general population and patient populations differ. Indeed, some studies supported this assumption (Froberg and Kane, 1989; Boyd et al., 1990; Llewellyn-Thomas et al., 1982; Zethraeus et al., 1999). For example, it was found that patients who have received colostomies rate the utility of alive with a stoma as much higher than those who do not experience colostomies (Boyd et al., 1990).

Chapter 3
The Impact of Diabetes on Health-State Utilities

However, some other studies (Pickard et al., 2013; Llewellyn-Thomas et al., 1984; Balaban et al., 1986; Dolders et al., 2006) including a meta-analysis (Dolders et al., 2006) found no or minimal difference in health-state utilities from general and patient populations, suggesting that the source of utility values may not be crucial.

The EQ-5D-3L is a standardized instrument that is widely used to measure the utility of health technologies for calculating quality-adjusted life years in economic evaluations (Dolan, 1997). It defines a total of 243 unique health states whose utility values are determined using the time trade-off (TTO) or visual analog scale (VAS) methods from general population samples. While the EQ-5D-3L has been recommended by many health technology assessment agencies for use in economic evaluations, it is not known whether its value sets based on the general populations' health preferences are suitable for clinical decision making where patients' preferences are most appropriate. The key question is: are the values of the EQ-5D-3L health states the same to the general population and the patients of interest? If they are the same or the difference is negligible, the EQ-5D-3L and its current value sets can be used to inform clinical decision making as well; otherwise, the values of the EQ-5D-3L health states from patients of interest should be used. A few studies compared the values of EQ-5D-3L health states to healthy individuals and unhealthy individuals showed mixed results. Pickard et al suggested that chronic conditions have trivial impact on utility values(2013); others suggested that patient and the general population have significantly different utility values (Suarez and Conner, 2001; Badia et al., 1996; Badia et al., 1998, De Wit et al., 2000; Mann et al., 2009).

The aim of our study was to compare the TTO values of EQ-5D-3L health states directly elicited from patients with type 2 diabetes mellitus (T2DM) and the general population to determine whether the values differed, and if so, how they differed.

3.2 Methods

3.2.1 Study participants

Consecutive outpatients with T2DM were approached and enrolled from the diabetes clinic of the National University Hospital from May to December 2012. The inclusion criteria are: 1) a diagnosis of type 2 diabetes mellitus; 2) Singapore citizens/Singapore permanent residents aged 21 years or above; 3) ability to read and converse in English. Consenting T2DM patients were interviewed by a trained interviewer to value 5 EQ-5D-3L health states in the clinic after their routine consultations.

A valuation study of the EQ-5D-3L health states in Singapore provided valuation data for EQ-5D-3L health states from a sample of the general Singaporean population. The sampling and recruitment procedures used were reported in detail in Chapter 4. Briefly, a random sample of non-institutional adult Singaporean residents were recruited and interviewed face-to-face in their homes by a trained interviewer. Each participant was asked to value a total of 10 EQ-5D-3L health states. Only the participants who valued the same EQ-5D-3L health states as T2DM patients did and who reported having no DM were included in the present study.

3.2.2 Survey procedures

An identical interview protocol was used to survey T2DM patients and in the general population study to measure the utilities of the EQ-5D-3L health states. The survey started with an example TTO task in which the interviewer demonstrated how the TTO tasks would be conducted using a time board and cards. Five states were presented to T2DM patients in a random order for valuation T2DM patients' own health status and demographic characteristics

Chapter 3
The Impact of Diabetes on Health-State Utilities

were assessed after the TTO valuation tasks.

In TTO tasks, each state was valued by asking a participant to state preferences for 11 questions each asking the participant's preference for two hypothetical lives: (a) living in the health state for 10 years and then die and (b) living in full health for x years and then die. The x values were integers ranging from 0 to 10, with one integer corresponding to one question. For each question, the response could be (a), (b), or equal preference (no preference). As previous studies found that TTO values are affected by the starting point of x values (Samuelsen et al., 2012), two starting points, 0 and 10 years, were used in the valuation tasks and were randomly assigned to each participant in our study. For each health state, half of the T2DM patients started with a question asking them to compare 0 year of full health (i.e. immediate death) to 10 years of life in the health state and the length of full health in subsequent questions was increased to 10 years by a step of 1 year (i.e. the bottom-up sequence); the other half of the T2DM patients started with comparing 10 years of full heath to 10 years of life in the health state and then the length of full health was decreased to 0 year with a step of 1 year (i.e. the top-down sequence).

If a T2DM patient preferred (b) when the x value was 0 (i.e. immediate death), another 11 questions would be given to the respondents for stating preferences, each question asking respondents' preference of two options: (a) living in full health for 10 years followed by 10 years in the health state and then die and (b) living in full health for y years and then die. The y values were also integers ranging from 0 to 10 and the values varied from 10 to 0 in all interviews. A time board and health-state cards were used as visual aids to help respondents comprehend the different life scenarios.

Both T2DM patients and participants from the general population received a gift voucher worth $20 on completion of the survey.

3.2.3 Health states valued

The health states valued in this study was defined by the EQ-5D-3L classification system which comprises 5 domains (i.e. mobility, self-care, usual activities, pain or discomfort, and anxiety or depression), with each domain having 3 functional levels: "no problems" (level 1); "some problems" (level 2); and "extreme problems" (level 3). EQ-5D-3L health states can be expressed using a five-digit code, with each digit representing the functional level of one domain. For example, a state in which a person has no problems in mobility and self-care, moderate problems in usual activities, moderate pain or discomfort, and extreme anxiety or depression can be coded as 11223. In this study, 3 mild(11112, 21112, and 21122), 4 severe(11223, 23221, 21231, and 23211), and 3 very severe(23332, 32322, and 33333) health states were selected to represent various severities. As valuing all 10 health states might be too burdensome to T2DM patients, we divided the 10 states into two blocks: 11112, 21112, 21231, 23221, and 32322 in one block; and 21122, 11223, 23211, 23332, and 33333 in the other block and randomly assigned each T2DM patient to value one block of health states. The EQ-5D-3L health states were divided into three categories: mild, moderate, and severe. One or two states were randomly selected from each category to construct a block of 5 states.

3.2.4 Data analysis

The TTO value for each health state was calculated for each participant who valued that health state. For health state considered as better than death, the TTO value was $x^*/10$, in which x^* is the x value at which equal preference was stated. If there were multiple x values, x^* was the mean of the values; if there was no value at which equal preference was stated, x^* was mean of the maximum value at which option (a) was preferred and the

Chapter 3
The Impact of Diabetes on Health-State Utilities

minimum value at which option (b) was preferred. For example, if at 0 to 5 years option (a) is preferred and at 6 to 10 years option (b) is preferred, the TTO value of the health state would be $[(5+6)/2]/10 = 0.55$. Similarly, the TTO value of a health state considered as worse than death is given by $(y^* - 10)/10$. Poor data quality was considered if a T2DM patient (or a participant from the general population) rated all 5 (10) health states as having the same value or worse than death. Data of poor quality was excluded from further analysis.

Data collected from T2DM patients and the general population sample was pooled for analysis. The characteristics of the two samples were compared using Chi-square tests.

Separate linear regression models were used to investigate the difference in TTO values of all health states, mild health states (i.e. 11112, 21112, and 21122), severe health problems (i.e. 11223, 23221, 21231, 23211, 23332, 32322, and 33333), and each of the health states between T2DM patients and the general population sample. In all models, the TTO value was regressed on the source of the value (T2DM patients or general population) with and without the adjustment of other factors. The factors adjusted for included age, gender, race, education, as well as the characteristics of the 10 EQ-5D-3L health states being valued whenever appropriate. All factors were coded into dummy variables and the random effects estimator was used in the models whenever appropriate to account for individual clustering of data.

3.3 Results

A total of 120 T2DM patients were recruited and interviewed in the study. After excluding patients whose TTO values were either the same ($n = 2$) or negative for all the 5 health states they valued ($n = 9$), 109 T2DM patients were used for comparison analysis. Fifty-two participants without

DM in the general population study valued the same health states valued by the T2DM patients. After excluding 4 participants valuing all states as worse than death and 2 participants rating all 10 states the same, 46 participants were included in the analysis. Compared to the general population, T2DM patients were more likely to be male, elder, non-Chinese, and better educated (Table 3.1).

Table 3.1 Characteristics of participants

	N(%)		P value
	T2DM patients	General population	
Gender			0.0029
Male	62(56.9)	23(50.0)	
Female	47(43.1)	23(50.0)	
Age group, years			<0.0001
21-60 years	71(65.1)	35(76.1)	
>60 years	38(34.9)	11(23.9)	
Education level			0.0007
College and higher	21(19.3)	6(13.0)	
Middle school and lower	88(80.7)	40(87.0)	
Race			<0.0001
Chinese	54(49.5)	28(60.9)	
non-Chinese	55(50.5)	18(39.1)	
H_bA1c level			
H_bA1c<6.5%	16(14.7)		
H_bA1c≥6.5%	87(85.3)		
Chronic conditions other than diabetes			<0.0001
Yes	40(36.7)	11(23.9)	
No	69(63.3)	35(76.1)	

T2DM: type 2 diabetes mellitus

All 10 health states considered, the mean TTO value was 0.04 and −0.02 for the T2DM patients and the general population sample, respectively ($P = 0.1643$). After adjusting for, however, T2DM patients' TTO value was 0.02 point lower than the general population sample ($P = 0.6527$). With and without adjustment of other variables, the mean TTO value of the general

Chapter 3
The Impact of Diabetes on Health-State Utilities

population sample was significantly lower than that of T2DM patients for mild health states. The mean difference (95% confidence interval [95% CI]) between the general population sample and T2DM patients was −0.15(−0.24, −0.06) before adjustment and −0.13(−0.25, −0.02) after adjustment. On the other hand, with and without adjustment, T2DM patients and the general population sample had similar mean TTO values for severe health states (Table 3.2). Hence, the difference in the means was greater for the T2DM patients than the general population sample.

Table 3.2 TTO values between T2DM patients and the general population

	T2DM patients	General population	Difference between T2DM patients and general population*	
	Mean (SD)	Mean (SD)	Unadjusted(95%CI)	Adjusted(95%CI)
All health states†	0.04(0.74)	−0.02(0.75)	−0.06(−0.16, 0.03)	0.02(−0.12, 0.15)
States without severe problems‡	0.64(0.31)	0.48(0.50)	−0.15(−0.24, −0.06)	−0.13(−0.25, −0.02)
States with severe problems‡	−0.24(0.73)	−0.24(0.71)	0.001(−0.11, 0.11)	0.02(−0.16, 0.19)

T2DM: type 2 diabetes mellitus; SD: standard deviation; CI: confidence interval; OR: odds ratio
* Reference group is T2DM patients and the random effect was used in the comparison analyses with and without adjustment
† Random effect linear regression model, in which age, gender, education, ethnicity, and the 10 EQ-5D-3L health states are adjusted
‡ Adjusted for age group, gender, education, and ethnicity only

The mean values of individual health states varied from −0.75 (for 33333) to 0.76 (for 11112) for T2DM patients and from −0.62 (for 33333) to 0.61 (for 11112) for the general population (Figure 3.1), with the range being 1.51 and 1.23 for T2DM patients and the general population sample, respectively. With and without adjustment, T2DM patients had systematically higher TTO values for mild health states. On the other hand, there was no systematic difference in the mean values between T2DM patients and the general population sample for severe health states (Figure 3.1).

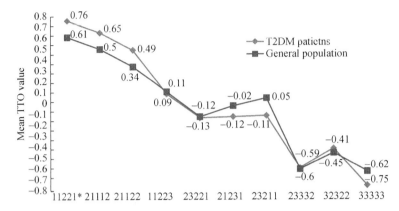

Figure 3.1　Mean TTO values for each of the 10 EQ-5D-3L health states between T2DM patients and the general population

* Difference in TTO values between T2DM patients and the general population is statistically significant with adjustment of age, gender, education, and ethnicity

3.4　Discussion

We found that the values of EQ-5D-3L states with mild health problems to T2DM patients were higher than to the general population, although the EQ-5D-3L states with severe health problems values were similarly undesirable to these two populations and as a result there was no significant difference between the two populations when all EQ-5D-3L health states were considered. Overall similarities in TTO values of EQ-5D-3L health states between patient and general populations were also observed in two previous studies. Pickard et al(2013)found that chronic conditions including DM have a negligible impact on TTO valuation in the general US population; Suarez Almazor and Conner Spady(2001)found that patients with rheumatoid arthritis and the general population have similar TTO values of 2 EQ-5D-3L health states. Also, our finding that T2DM patients rated mild health states better than the general population is consistent with findings from two previous studies (Badia et al., 1998; De Wit et al., 2000); however, in both of those studies, patients also rated severe EQ-5D-3L states as better than the general population, which is inconsistent with the finding about severe EQ-5D-3L health problems in our study. The relatively higher or similar EQ-5D-3L values of patients to non-patients may be explained by the prospect theory (Treadwell and Lenert, 1999). According to this theory, valuation of hypothetical health states is affected by a rater's own health status. As a result, a health state is perceived as similarly valuable by patients and healthy persons if their health status are similar or if the health state to be valued is far better or worse than the health status of patients or non-patients; on the other hand, if patients and non-patients have different health status and the health states to be valued are not very different from their health status, patients have higher valuation than non-patients. It should be noted that the prospect theory is not supported by some studies (Feeny and Eng, 2005; Wittenberg et al., 2005). The mixed results from the comparisons of patients and general populations may also be due to the different valuation methods (i.e. TTO and VAS) or elicitation procedure (e.g. mode of administration, search procedures, the use of visual aid, etc) (Dolan et al., 1996; Attema et al., 2013) used in those studies.

Our result suggests that the utility gain associated with a transition from a mild health state to a severe health state is greater to T2DM patients than to the general population. For example, according to our study, the utility gain from a transition between 23332 and 21122 would be 1.08 and 0.94 to T2DM patients and the general population, respectively. This means for a health intervention which can achieve such an improvement in health is more attractive according to patients' preferences than the general populations' preferences. This implication of our results is consistent with that from some previous studies (Lenert et al., 1999; Nord, 1995; Ratcliffe et al., 2007; Fujiikee et al., 2011) but inconsistent with that from some other studies (Suarez and Conner, 2001; Badia et al., 1996; Badia et al., 1998, De Wit et al., 2000). This is not surprising as the relative health-state values elicited from patients and the general population or non-patients differed and varied with the severity of the health states to be valued. Given these mixed findings, it might be worthwhile to determine the values of the EQ-5D-3L health states to patients with a certain condition. Such disease-specific EQ-5D-3L value sets, if more sensitive to treatment benefit than the conventional value sets, should be used in studies to inform clinical decision making for the relevant disease.

Our study has two limitations. First, in the study, each health state was only rated by approximately 60 T2DM patients and 50 members of the general population, which may impair the statistical power. Second, the cases and controls were not matched in terms of age, gender, education and race. Nevertheless, we adjusted these factors in the analysis to account for their influence. Third, we only recruited outpatients with T2DM, the findings may not be generalized to inpatients with T2DM who may have more severe health problems.

In conclusion, our study indicates that the utility values of mild EQ-5D-3L health states are higher to T2DM patients than to the general population and therefore the EQ-5D-3L values based on the general population's preferences could be insensitive and underestimate the effectiveness of health inventions for T2DM. How the values of EQ-5D-3L health states to patients and the general population differ warrant further investigation.

Chapter 4

Valuation of EQ-5D-3L Health States in Singapore

4.1 Introduction

Quality adjusted life years (QALYs) that combines both quantity and quality of life is the outcome measure in cost-utility analysis (CUA) (Torrance, 1986). To calculate QALYs, health-state utility that indicates the relative value of health states using a 0 (being dead) to 1.0 (full health) scale should be used as the quality-of-life weight (Torrance, 1986). Health-state utility values elicited from the general population are typically used in CUA when the purpose of the analysis is to inform decision making in allocation of healthcare resources (Dolan, 1999). Health-state utility can be measured using valuation techniques such as time trade-off (TTO) (Torrance et al., 1972) and standard gamble (SG) (Torrance, 1986). However, those methods are difficult to administer and cognitively demanding to respondents. Alternatively, preference-based instruments such as the EQ-5D-3L (Dolan, 1997), the health utilities index (HUI) (Feeny et al., 2002), and the short form 6-dimensions ($SF-6D_{36}$) (Brazier et al., 2002) can be used to obtain health-state utility values much more easily. Those instruments classify a person's health into one of a series of predefined health states whose utility values are already known.

The preference-based EQ-5D-3L instrument includes two parts: a health-state classification system and a value set comprising the utility values of all the health states defined by the classification system. The EQ-5D-3L classification system consists of 5 domains: mobility, self-care, usual activities, pain/discomfort, and anxiety/depression, with each domain being described as three levels: "no problems" (level 1); "some problems" (level 2); and "severe problems" (level 3). Each health state described by EQ-5D-3L can be coded into a five-digit number. For example, a health state in which a person has no problems in mobility and self-care, no pain or discomfort, but moderate problems in usual activities and severe anxiety or depression can be coded as 11213. This classification system defines a total of 243 (3^5) unique health states and can be used as a questionnaire for respondents to classify their own health status. The first value set for the EQ-5D-3L health states was derived from the general UK population in the measurement and valuation of health (MVH) study using a TTO method in 1997 (Dolan, 1997). Country-specific EQ-5D-3L value sets were subsequently developed using a similar research protocol in many other countries (Shaw et al., 2007; Lee et al., 2009; Tsuchiya et al., 2002; Tongsiri and Cairns, 2011; Yusof et al., 2012; Golicki et al., 2010; Jelsma et al., 2002; Lamers et al., 2006; Cleemput, 2010; Wittrup-Jensen, 2002). Studies showed that utility values of EQ-5D-3L health states differed across countries (Tongsiri and Cairns, 2011; Jelsma et al., 2003; Wittrup-Jensen, 2002; Norman et al., 2009), suggesting that each country should develop its own value set for using the EQ-5D-3L in economic evaluations of health technologies.

In Singapore, the EQ-5D-3L questionnaire has been psychometrically validated (Luo et al., 2003a; Luo et al., 2003b; Luo et al., 2003c; Luo et al., 2009; Gao et al., 2009) and widely used in clinical and epidemiological studies (Abdin et al., 2010; Wang et al., 2012; Chong et al., 2012; Zhang et al., 2009). However, the values of the EQ-5D-3L health states to Singaporeans are not known. As a result, researchers using the EQ-5D-3L in Singapore had to use the UK, US, or Japanese value set to acquire utility

Chapter 4
Valuation of EQ-5D-3L Health States in Singapore

scores (Luo et al., 2003a; Luo et al., 2003b; Luo et al., 2003c; Luo et al., 2009; Gao et al., 2009; Abdin et al., 2010; Wang et al., 2012; Chong et al., 2012; Zhang et al., 2009). The aim of this study was therefore to derive a Singapore societal value set for EQ-5D-3L health states using the TTO method.

4.2 Methods

4.2.1 Sampling and recruitment

This study was approved by the National University of Singapore Institutional Review Board (NUS-IRB). In the study, we drew a nationally representative sample of the non-institutionalized general Singaporean population. We excluded the institutionalized population because our purpose was to estimate the general population's health preferences which are most relevant to decision making in health resource allocation (Gold et al., 1996). A three-stage sampling method was used to recruit 500 residents aged 21 years and above, with quotas set to achieve similarity between the sample and the general adult Singaporean population in age, gender, and housing type (an indicator of socio-economic status). The two minority ethnic groups (i.e. Malays and Indians) were oversampled and only the English-speaking Singaporeans were recruited. The sampling procedure was as follows. First, a total of 20 locations were randomly selected from a sampling frame comprising over 9,000 residential locations, covering almost all public housing blocks in Singapore. Second, 25 households were recruited from each selected location using a systematic sampling method. Third, one resident from each consenting household was invited to the study. If the household had more than one eligible resident, the first one whom interviewer approached was recruited. Residents who were foreign workers or could not speak English were excluded. All respondents were interviewed face-to-face in their homes by a trained interviewer. Respondents received a gift voucher worths $20 on completion of the interview.

4.2.2 The valuation interview

The interview started with an assessment of the respondent's health status using the EQ-5D-3L questionnaire. This was for familiarizing the respondent with the EQ-5D-3L descriptive system. Before proceeding to valuation of the EQ-5D-3L health states, the interviewer went through an example TTO task with the respondent to make sure the latter understand the questions. The interviewer then showed 10 EQ-5D-3L health states, one at a time in a random order, to the respondent and conducted the valuation tasks as described below. The respondent's demographic characteristics and feedback on the interview were collected after the completion of the valuation tasks.

In each valuation task, the TTO value of a health state was elicited by asking a respondent to state preferences for 11 pairs of scenarios each comprising two options: (a) to live in the health state for 10 years and then die; and (b) to live in full health for x years and then die. The values for x were integers ranging from 0 to 10. For each pair of the scenarios, the response could be (a), (b), or equal preference (no preference). As previous studies found that TTO values are affected by the starting point of x values (Samuelsen et al., 2012), two starting points, 0 and 10 years, were used in the valuation tasks and were randomly assigned to each participant in our study. For each health state, half of the respondents start with a question asking them to compare 0 year of full health (i.e. immediate death) with 10 years of life in the health state and the length of full health in subsequent questions was increased to 10 years each time by 1 year (i.e. the bottom-up sequence); the other half of the respondents start with 10 years of full health with 10 years of life in the health state and then the length of full health was

Chapter 4
Valuation of EQ-5D-3L Health States in Singapore

decreased to 0 year by a step of 1 year (i.e. the top-down sequence).

If a respondent's preference was (b) when the x value was 0 (i.e. immediate death), another 11 pairs of scenarios would be posed to the respondent for stating preferences, each pair comprising two options: (a) to live in full health for 10 years followed by 10 years in the health state and then die; and (b) to live in full health for y years and then die. The values for y were integers ranging from 0 to 10 and the values were used in the order from 10 to 0 in all interviews. As in previous EQ-5D-3L valuation studies (Dolan, 1997; Shaw et al., 2007), a time board and show cards were used as visual aids to help respondents comprehend the different life scenarios.

4.2.3 The health states

A total of 80 EQ-5D-3L health states were included in the study for valuation. Those included state 33333 and 79 states that we selected through reviewing primary EQ-5D-3L data collected in past surveys of general and patient populations. Using pre-defined definitions, 24, 32, and 24 of the selected health states fell into the category of mild, moderate, and severe health states, respectively. Mild states had no domain in level 3 and up to three domains in level 2, severe states had at least two domains in level 3, and all other states were considered moderate. The 80 health states were stratified and randomly distributed into 8 blocks, with each block comprising 3 mild, 4 moderate, and 3 severe states (Table 4.1). Arrangements were made such that each block of health states were rated by similar number of respondents.

Table 4.1 Health states valued in the study

Severity	Block A	Block B	Block C	Block D	Block E	Block F	Block G	Block H
Mild	21121	21122	12122	11221	21212	12212	12121	11222
	22112	11112	12221	11211	12111	12211	22121	11122
	22211	21112	11121	21221	21211	21111	11212	22111

(To be continued)

Measuring Health-State Utilities for Cost-Utility Analysis
测量健康效用以用于成本效用分析

(Continued)

Severity	Block A	Block B	Block C	Block D	Block E	Block F	Block G	Block H
Moderate	32221	23221	22212	22222	11232	21222	21131	12231
	11132	21231	13221	23222	22221	21113	12223	12222
	11123	11223	21312	21232	22311	11113	22223	11131
	21223	23211	22321	12232	21322	21321	11213	21311
Severe	33323	32322	21233	22331	33222	13332	23322	33312
	22323	23332	12332	23312	33311	13333	33321	11233
	23232	33333	33331	23333	23311	23323	33332	32332

4.3 Statistical analysis

4.3.1 Calculation of TTO values

The TTO value of each health state was estimated for each respondent who valued that health state as follows. If the health state was considered better than death, the value was given by $X/10$, where X is the x value at which equal preference was stated. If there are multiple x values, X is the mean of the values; if there is no value at which equal preference was stated, X is mean of the maximum value at which option (a) was preferred and the minimum value at which option (b) was preferred. For example, if at 0 to 5 years option (a) is preferred and at 6 to 10 years option (b) is preferred, the TTO value of the health state would be $[(5+6)/2]/10 = 0.55$. Similarly, the TTO value of a health state considered as worse than death is given by $(Y-10)/10$. Poor data quality was considered if a respondent rated all 10 health states as having the same value or worse than death, or rated only two or fewer health states. Data of poor quality was excluded from modeling analysis.

4.3.2 Modeling of TTO values

Linear regression models using various functional forms were tested with the TTO data. Consistent with previous studies (Dolan, 1997; Shaw et al., 2007), model inputs were characteristics of the health states only and disutility (i.e. 1 minus TTO value) of the health states was modeled. The functional forms we tested included the main-effects, N3, and D1 models. The main-effects model contained 10 dummy variables, including M2 and M3 for mobility, S2 and S3 for self-care, U2 and U3 for usual activities, P2 and P3 for pain/discomfort, and A2 and A3 for anxiety/depression. Since each domain was described using three different levels, two dummy variables were needed. The N3 model is the main-effects model with addition of a dummy variable N3. The N3 term takes the value of 1 if any domain of a health state is in level 3; otherwise the value is 0 (Dolan, 1997). Both the main-effects and N3 models were estimated with and without a constant in our study. Without the constant, the models assume no disutility for state 11111, which is consistent with the expected utility theory and was recommended (Brazier et al., 2002). The D1 model contains the D1, and I2, I22, I3 and I32 terms in addition to the 10 main effects (Shaw et al., 2007). The D1 term represents the number of domains at level 2 or level 3 minus 1; the I2 term is the number of domains at level 2 minus 1; the I3 term is the number of domains at level 3 minus 1; the I22 and the I32 terms are squared I2 and I3 terms, respectively. The D1 model does not contain the constant term as the D1 term is a pseudo constant term. Hence, a total of 5 different functional forms were tested: (1) main effects with a constant; (2) main effects without a constant; (3) main effects with a constant and the N3 term; (4) main effects with the N3 term only; and (5) main effects with D1 and related terms

All functional forms were estimated using the TTO data at both individual and aggregate levels. At individual level, the assumption of independence for the ordinary-least square (OLS) estimator was violated since each respondent valued multiple health states. For this reason the random effects (RE) model and the fixed effects (FE) estimators were also used. The Lagrange Multiplier (LM) test (Silvey, 1959) was used to test the model assumption for OLS versus RE or FE models, and the Hausman test (Hausman, 1978) was used to compare the appropriateness of the RE and FE models. At aggregate level, the disutility of the 80 health states (calculated as 1 minus the mean TTO value) was modeled using the OLS estimator. All models were tested for heteroskedasticity using the Breusch-Pagan test (Breusch and Pagan, 1979) and normality of residuals using Shaprio-Wilk test (Shapiro and Wilk, 1965).

4.3.3 Evaluation of model performance

Four criteria were used to determine which model had the best performance and therefore should be selected to predict the EQ-5D-3L values. Those were, in the order of high to low priority, consistency, bias, precision, and parsimony. Consistency requires the predictions for measured and unmeasured EQ-5D-3L states to be consistent with the utility theory. That means that more severe problems (e.g. "extreme pain/discomfort") should be associated with more disutility than less severe problems (e.g. "moderate pain/discomfort") and that worse health states (e.g. 11133) should have lower TTO values than better health states (e.g. 11132). While assessment of prediction consistency can be based on the estimated regression coefficients for the main-effects and N3 models, it is not straightforward for the D1 model because of its complex model specification. We therefore compared D1 model predicted values for all possible pairs of EQ-5D-3L health states. Prediction bias refers to systematically higher or lower predictions than observed values. We were particularly concerned about prediction bias for very mild and very severe health states. For assessing prediction bias, we examined the overall agreement between predicted and observed mean TTO values for the 80 health states using intra-class correlation coefficient (ICC) (Fayers and

Machin, 2005). We also used the Bland-Altman plot (Bland and Altman, 1986) to visually assess the prediction bias in different segments of the utility scale. Prediction precision of the models was evaluated in terms of mean absolute error (MAE), the numbers of prediction errors greater than $|0.10|$ and $|0.20|$. Lastly, if multiple models performed similarly in consistency, bias, and precision, the model using the simplest functional form would be preferred (i.e. model parsimony).

In both individual-level and aggregate-level modeling analysis, sampling weights were applied to the data to reflect the distributions of age, gender, and ethnicity of the general adult Singaporean population in 2010 (Department of Statistic Singapore, 2013). Analyses were performed with SAS 9.2 and STATA 12.0.

4.4 Results

4.4.1 Respondents' characteristics

A total of 505 respondents were successfully interviewed, representing a response rate of 46.8%. After excluding respondents whose TTO scores were either the same ($n = 2$) or negative for all the 10 health states they rated ($n = 47$), data from 456 respondents was used for modeling analysis. There were no significant differences in socio-demographics between excluded and included respondents, and characteristics of the included respondents were similar to those of the general adult Singaporean population except that by design there was a higher proportion of Malays (13.3%) and Indians (17.3%) in our sample (Table 4.2).

Measuring Health-State Utilities for Cost-Utility Analysis
测量健康效用以用于成本效用分析

Table 4.2 Socio-demographic statistics of full sample and valuation sample compared with Singapore population

Characteristics	N(%) Full sample (N = 505)	N(%) Valuation sample (N = 456)	P value*	Singapore population(%)
Citizenship				
Citizen	455(90.1)	409(89.6)	0.325	86.4
Permanent residence	50(9.9)	47(10.4)		13.6
Gender				
Male	247(48.9)	228(50.0)	0.199	49.2
Female	258(51.1)	228(50.0)		50.8
Ethnicity				
Chinese	339(67.1)	310(67.9)	0.475	74.2
Malay	70(14.0)	60(13.3)		13.3
Indian	88(17.4)	79(17.3)		9.2
Others	8(1.6)	7(1.6)		3.3
Age, years				
20–29	82(16.2)	78(17.0)	0.325	17.7
30–39	95(18.8)	88(19.3)		20.8
40–49	102(20.2)	89(19.5)		21.5
50–59	119(23.6)	106(23.2)		19.8
60 or more	107(21.4)	95(21.0)		20.2
Education level				
No formal education	8(1.6)	8(1.8)	0.328	19.6
Primary	50(10.0)	45(10.0)		12.1
Lower secondary	24(4.6)	19(4.0)		10.9
Secondary	142(27.7)	121(26.3)		24.6
Upper secondary	79(15.8)	74(16.4)		9.9
Polytechnic diploma	69(13.6)	67(14.4)		6.2
Other diploma	33(6.6)	29(6.4)		4.9
University	100(20.0)	94(20.8)		11.7
Working Status				
Working	324(66.3)	297(65.3)	0.412	Not available
Homemaker	73(14.4)	68(14.8)		
Student	25(5)	25(5.5)		
Full-time national service	6(1.2)	5(1.1)		
Unemployed	16(3.2)	13(2.9)		
Retired	51(10.0)	47(10.4)		
Chronic conditions				
Yes	145(28.7)	128(28.3)	0.500	Not available
No	360(71.3)	328(71.7)		
EQ-5D-3L				Not available
Mobility				
Some problems	83(16.6)	78(17.3)	0.189	

(To be continued)

(Continued)

Characteristics	N(%)		P value*	Singapore population(%)
	Full sample (N = 505)	Valuation sample (N = 456)		
Extreme problems	11(2.2)	11(2.4)		
Self-care				
Some problems	9(1.8)	8(1.8)	0.899	
Extreme problems	7(1.4)	7(1.6)		
Usual activities				
Some problems	19(3.8)	18(4.0)	0.484	
Extreme problems	11(2.2)	10(2.2)	0.939	
Pain / discomfort				
Some problems	119(23.8)	111(24.6)	0.179	
Extreme problems	20(4.0)	19(4.2)	0.451	
Anxiety / depression				
Some problems	33(6.6)	29(6.4)	0.614	
Extreme problems	5(1.0)	5(1.1)		

* comparison between valuation sample and excluded respondents

4.4.2 Distribution of TTO values

The 456 respondents generated a total of 4,538 TTO values for the 80 health states. The distribution of those TTO values was bimodal with mean being 0.09 (standard deviation: 0.809). Among the 4,538 values, 1,363 (29.9%) of them was −1, 138 of them was 0(3.0%), and 167(3.7%) of them was 1. Overall, there was no statistically significant difference in TTO values between participants who started the questions from 0 years (mean: 0.036) and those who started the questions from 10 years (mean: 0.152, $P = 0.2865$). In 47 of the 4,538 TTO tasks(1%) completed by 24 respondents, at least one indifference response was observed; multiple indifference responses were observed in 31 TTO tasks completed by 16 respondents.

4.4.3 Modeling analysis

Modeling of individual-level data showed that all the seven models fit the data reasonably well (Table 4.3). Regression coefficients for the 10 main effects in each model were statistically significant and consistent with the utility theory in that more severe health problems are associated with higher disutility. For example, level-2 mobility problems (M2) and level-3 mobility problems (M3) were associated with a disutility of 0.114 and 0.290, respectively, in the RE model including the main effects and the N3 term. As can be seen in Table 4.3, N3 and D1 models performed better than main-effects models in prediction bias measured by ICC and prediction precision measured by MAE. The LM test suggested that the RE and FE estimators were more appropriate than the OLS estimator ($P < 0.0001$ for all). The Hausman test indicated that the RE estimator was not as efficient as the FE estimator for all the model specifications ($P < 0.05$ for both). Predictions of all models using the individual-level data did not pass the Breusch-Pagan test for heteroskedasticity or Shaprio-Wilk test for normality of residuals ($P < 0.001$), suggesting certain degrees of model mis-specification.

Modeling results of the mean TTO scores for the 80 health states using the OLS estimator are displayed in Table 4.4. Regression coefficients estimated for the main effects, N3 and D1 terms were statistically significant and in the ranges as we expected. Similar to findings in individual-level modeling, the N3 and D1 models outperformed the main-effects models in prediction bias and precision. However, different from models based on individual-level data, all the models based on the aggregate data passed the Breusch-Pagan test for heteroschediscity and Shaprio-Wilk test for normality of residuals. For example, P-values of the two tests for N3 model without a constant were 0.327 and 0.510, respectively. Bland-Altman plots revealed that the N3 model without a constant generally did not suffer from prediction bias at any segments of the utility scale, while all other models predicted lower TTO values for health states with mild and/or severe health problems (Figure 4.1). The middle dotted lines stand for mean differences between actual and predicted scores; the upper and lower dotted lines stand for ± 1.96 standard deviation of the mean differences.

Chapter 4
Valuation of EQ-5D-3L Health States in Singapore

Table 4.3 Parameter estimates and goodness-of-fitness statistics at individual level using fixed effect (FE) and random effect (RE) regression

Variable	FE				RE		
	Main effect	N3	Main effect with constant	Main effect without constant	N3 with constant	N3 without constant	D1
Constant	0.1626	0.1059	0.1544		0.0978		
M2	0.0932	0.0856	0.1028	0.1352	0.0940	0.1135	0.2018
M3	0.2952	0.2759	0.3011	0.3204	0.2788	0.2898	0.5390
S2	0.1380	0.1619	0.1369	0.1588	0.1607	0.1751	0.2736
S3	0.3370	0.3049	0.3407	0.3487	0.3083	0.3119	0.5498
U2	0.2528	0.2058	0.2559	0.2840	0.2095	0.2249	0.3176
U3	0.4534	0.3163	0.4518	0.4673	0.3162	0.3202	0.5409
P2	0.1483	0.1306	0.1468	0.1757	0.1288	0.1458	0.2443
P3	0.3499	0.2294	0.3460	0.3768	0.2252	0.2392	0.4812
A2	0.1110	0.1323	0.1116	0.1336	0.1329	0.1472	0.2299
A3	0.3645	0.2694	0.3643	0.3884	0.2685	0.2794	0.5240
D1							−0.1148
I3square							−0.0456
N3		0.2816			0.2825	0.2940	
ICC	0.910	0.937	0.908	0.914	0.939	0.935	0.928
MAE	0.1334	0.1137	0.1326	0.1393	0.1125	0.1187	0.1288
No. (of 80)>0.1	42	37	43	37	38	43	40
No. (of 80)>0.2	18	15	17	21	13	14	19

All coefficients are statistically significantly at 0.05 confidence level

FE; fixed effect regressior; RE: random effect regression; M2: mobility level 2; M3: mobility level 3; S2: self-care level 2; S3: self-care level 3; U2: usual activities level 2; U3: usual activities level 3; P2: pain / discomfort level 2; P3: pain / discomfort level 3; A2: anxiety / depression level 2; A3: anxiety / depression level 3; D1: number of domains with problems beyond the first; I3square: the square term of I3 that is the number of domains at level 3 beyond the first; N3: any domains on level 3; ICC: intraclass correlation coefficient; MAE: mean absolute error

Measuring Health-State Utilities for Cost-Utility Analysis
测量健康效用以用于成本效用分析

Table 4.4 Parameter estimates and goodness-of-fitness statistics at aggregated level using OLS regression

Variable	Main effect with constant	Main effect without constant	N3 with constant	N3 without constant	D1
Constant	0.1335		0.0809		
M2	0.1558	0.2017	0.1419	0.1678	0.2658
M3	0.3280	0.3549	0.2906	0.3040	0.6961
S2	0.1160	0.1489	0.1409	0.1615	0.2485
S3	0.3826	0.3944	0.3421	0.3465	0.6493
U2	0.2730	0.3184	0.2316	0.2555	0.3649
U3	0.4240	0.4549	0.3099	0.3209	0.6115
P2	0.1469	0.1857	0.1249	0.1462	0.2529
P3	0.3289	0.3694	0.2125	0.2291	0.5716
A2	0.1080	0.1439	0.1280	0.1501	0.2376
A3	0.3563	0.3942	0.2620	0.2784	0.5219
D1					−0.1310
I3square					−0.0915
N3			0.2740	0.2905	
ICC	0.914	0.919	0.938	0.941	0.938
MAE	0.1324	0.1318	0.1125	0.1137	0.1153
No. (of 80)>0.1	45	42	37	35	34
No. (of 80)>0.2	17	15	13	13	14

All coefficients are statistically significantly at 0.05 confidence level

OLS: ordinary least square; M2: mobility level 2; M3: mobility level 3; S2: self-care level 2; S3: self-care level 3; U2: usual activities level 2; U3: usual activities level 3; P2: pain / discomfort level 2; P3: pain / discomfort level 3; A2: anxiety / depression level 2; A3: anxiety / depression level 3; D1: number of domains with problems beyond the first; I3square: the square term of I3 that is the number of domains at level 3 beyond the first; N3: any domains on level 3; ICC: intraclass correlation coefficient; MAE: mean absolute error

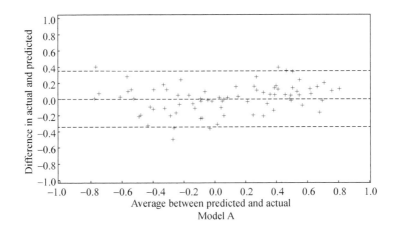

Model A

Chapter 4
Valuation of EQ-5D-3L Health States in Singapore

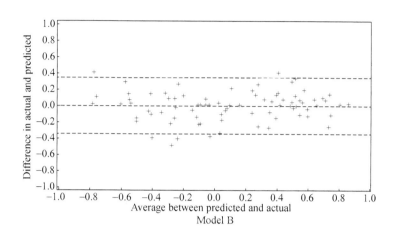
Model B

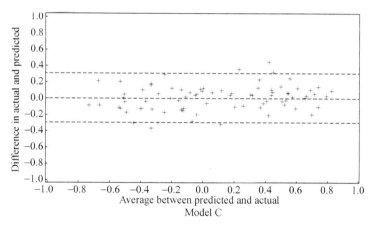
Model C

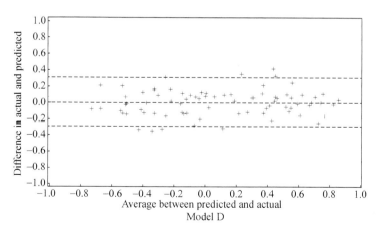
Model D

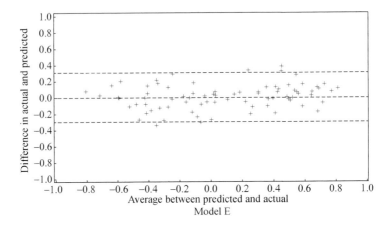

Figure 4.1　Bland-Altman plots of actual and predicted scores based on OLS regression at aggregated level

X axis is the average between actual and predicted scores; Y axis is the actual scores minus predicted scores. Model A: main effect model with a constant; Model B: main effect model without a constant; Model C: N3 model with a constant; Model D: N3 model without a constant; Model E: D1 model

4.5　Discussion

It is worth noting that the design of our study differs from that of past EQ-5D-3L valuation studies in several ways. First, health states considered worse than death were valued using the lead-time TTO method (Devlin et al., 2011) which allowed health states better and worse than death to be measured in the same timeframe, that is, 10 years. In MVH and other EQ-5D-3L valuation studies, states better and worse than death were valued using different time frames and scenarios. It should be noted that the lead-time TTO allows valuation of states better and worse than death using a uniform procedure (Devlin et al., 2011). However, we did not use the lead-time TTO to value states better than death because lead-time TTO resulted in low values for states better than death in a previous study (Luo et al., 2013). Another difference between lead-time and classic TTO procedures is data censoring. The negative value in our study and the MVH study was censored at −1.0 and −39, respectively. In the MVH study, all negative values were arbitrarily compressed to the range of −1.0 to 0; in contrast, we did not perform such data transformation. Therefore, the estimated values in our study and previous studies were not really comparable.

Second, we measured approximately one third of all the EQ-5D-3L health states which were observed in empirical studies. Most previous studies estimated the EQ-5D-3L value set based on only 42 directly measured health states (Dolan, 1997; Shaw et al., 2007; Yusof et al., 2012; Golicki et al., 2010; Jelsma et al., 2002; Lamers et al., 2006; Cleemput, 2010; Wittrup-Jensen, 2002). We think selecting health states observed in reality is more meaningful than selecting health states in order to evenly cover the whole space the descriptive system defines. This is because some of EQ-5D-3L health states are never or rarely observed in health surveys because those states are either implausible (e.g. 33111) or too severe (e.g. 33333). Valuation of those rarely observed health states would be difficult to respondents and the values of those states are less useful. Therefore, we selected health states by reviewing primary EQ-5D-3L data collected from various populations. By directly valuing approximately one third of the 243 EQ-5D-3L health states, we substantially reduce the interpolation space for estimating the value set. Theoretically, the smaller the interpolation space, the smaller the prediction bias (i.e. systematic error) for the unobserved health states would be. Nevertheless, the increase of the number of health states was at the cost of decreasing the number of observations for each health state, given that the sample size and the number of health states each participant valued were fixed. As a result, the prediction precision (i.e. random error) for the observed health states was impaired (see below for more discussion on prediction precision).

Third, we asked all respondents to state preferences for the same set of health scenarios in each TTO task and posed those scenarios to respondents in two different orders. In contrast, TTO tasks stopped as soon as respondents indicated indifference and each TTO task began with a scenario of 5 years of full health in the MVH study. A recent study showed that respondents tend to state indifference within the first few TTO questions (Luo et al., 2013) and an experiment in Norway found association between TTO values and the starting points of the iteration procedure (Samuelsen et al., 2012). Therefore, we required our respondents to consider the full range of scenarios even they stated indifference in the beginning of the iteration process. Using this design, we minimized premature responses and forced respondents to think more thoroughly about their answers. A previous study found that some respondents form their responses during the valuation tasks rather than knowing their indifference points before the tasks (Brazier, 2007). We did not find a significant difference in TTO values between respondents using different starting points, suggesting that our study was free from the starting point bias.

Our modeling results suggest that the N3 model without a constant estimated using the aggregate data should be recommended for generating the EQ-5D-3L health states in Singapore. Our modeling results are consistent with those in previous studies in several ways. First, aggregated data achieved better modeling results than individual data. Two previous EQ-5D-3L valuation studies also recommended a model based on aggregated data for the same reasons — models based on individual-level data did not pass the tests for model misspecification (Lee et al., 2009; Liu et al., 2012). Those two studies directly measured approximately 100 EQ-5D-3L states which are not exactly same as those measured in our study. Other studies measured only 42 or fewer states and therefore did not perform aggregate level modeling. However, model misspecification was also observed in some of those studies (Dolan, 1997; Shaw et al., 2007; Lee et al., 2009; Wittrup-Jensen et al., 2002). Second, models with the N3 term outperformed those without the term, which was the result in most of the previous EQ-5D-3L valuation studies (Dolan, 1997; Lee et al., 2009; Yusof et al., 2012; Golicki et al., 2010; Lamers et al., 2006; Cleemput et al., 2010; Wittrup-Jensen et al., 2002). Third, the model without a constant fit the data better than those with a constant. Although no EQ-5D-3L valuation studies so far recommended such a model specification, Brazier et al. recommended a similar model specification in a study of SG values for SF-6D$_{36}$ health states (2002). The decision was based on both utility theory and the modeling results. The existence of a positive constant means the value for full health is lower than 1.0, which is against the utility theory and therefore suggests the valuation method is not optimal. Our study found that the existence of the constant would lead to underestimated values especially for mild health states. It is not known whether the same effect exists in previous studies and therefore future studies are needed to further investigate the implications of the constant in the modeling of health-state utility values.

On the other hand, the results of our study were markedly different from those from previous studies in two aspects. One noticeable difference is that the values of EQ-5D-3L health states to Singaporeans are lower than those to all other populations. A total of 145 (59.7%) EQ-5D-3L states were considered worse than death by Singaporeans, with the lowest value being -0.769 (for state 33333). In contrast, 84, 8, and 6 EQ-5D-3L states have a negative value according to the utility function developed in the UK (Dolan, 1997), Korea (Lee et al., 2009), and Japan (Tsuchiya et al., 2002), respectively. The low TTO values could be partially explained by data collection and analysis procedures. First of all, as we previously discussed, all other EQ-5D-3L valuation studies perform data transformation for negative values but we did not do it.

Also, the duration for all health states was 10 years in our study while in all other studies the duration for states worse than death was less than 10 years. Evidence showed that severe health states are less preferred if they are in longer durations (Stalmeier et al., 2007). We suspect that this was the main reason for marked censoring effects in our study. In the meanwhile, we could not exclude the possibility that Singaporeans do not mind to die or die sooner in order to avoid severe poor health problems than people in other countries. Indeed, Singaporeans valued EQ-5D-5L health states as less desirable than the people in China (Luo et al., 2013). The reason might be the concern about healthcare costs which are mainly borne by individuals in Singapore. A recent study found that Singaporean cancer patients would not choose to use better but more expensive treatment if they had to pay for it (BMJ Group Blogs, 2013).

Another major difference between our study and previous studies was model fit. Model fit in our study was poorer than that in previous studies. The MAE of all the models in our study was > 0.10 while the MAE in previous studies ranged from 0.02 (Tsuchiya et al., 2002) to 0.08 (Tongsiri, et al., 2011). The poorer model prediction precision was unlikely due to the large number of health states valued because the MAE in a Korean study (states valued: 101) (Lee et al., 2009) and a Chinese study (states valued: 97) (Liu et al., 2012) was less than 0.03. The poorer prediction precision of our models was an indication of greater data variability which should be the joint effects of several design factors. First, multiple starting points in the valuation exercise should have resulted in greater variance in data. TTO values were found to be associated with the starting point (Samuelsen et al., 2012). Different from our study, all previous EQ-5D-3L valuation studies followed the MVH protocol to use a single starting point. Second, we used a relatively small number of respondents to value a large number of health states. As a result, each health state was only rated by approximately 60 respondents. Third, we did not transform negative values as investigators of previous studies. The transformation performed in other studies compressed data distribution and variability.

The main limitation of the study was the small number of observations for each health state. It should have contributed to the relative poor prediction precision of our models. However, the small number of observations per state allowed valuation of 80 health states which reduced the interpolation space and the predication bias for unobserved health states. Another limitation of our study was inclusion of English-speaking Singaporeans only. Due to limited resources, we excluded Singaporeans who can not speak English. It should be noted that it is important to use a representative sample in such a valuation study. However, English is the primary language of academic education in Singapore and about 80% of the total Singapore population can speak English (Pakir, 1999). In addition, another study which is currently under way comparing health-state preference values across subgroups of Singaporeans found that survey language may not have significant impact on health-state preferences. Lastly, we did not ask respondents to rank and rate the health states before the TTO tasks as previous studies. The ranking and rating exercises may familiarize the participants with those health states and result in more accurate TTO values.

In conclusion, the time trade-off value set for the EQ-5D-3L can be estimated using the modeling approach in the multi-cultural, multi-ethnic Singapore. Although the estimation precision is not optimal, domestic preference values for EQ-5D-3L health states are preferred to foreign values for conducting cost-utility analysis in Singapore.

Chapter 5

Predicting Preference-Based SF-6D$_{36}$ Index Scores from the SF-8 Health Survey

5.1 Introduction

Cost-utility analysis (CUA) is increasingly used when a decision-maker evaluates a potentially more effective, yet more expensive intervention or health technology (Drummond et al., 2005; Bloom, 2004). In such economic evaluations, the effectiveness outcome is often measured as life-years weighted by health-state utilities, or quality-adjusted life-years (QALYs). The preference-based health-status instrument is a convenient approach to obtain health-state utility scores. Examples of preference-based measures include the quality of wellbeing scale (QWB) (Patrick and Erickson, 1993), the EQ-5D-3L (Dolan, 1996), the health utilities index (HUI) (Feeny et al., 2002), and the Short Form 6-dimensions (SF-6D$_{36}$) (Brazier et al., 2002) which is a multi-attribute health classification system developed from the short form 36 health survey (SF-36) (Ware et al., 1993).

It is common that researchers who want to conduct CUA find the available effectiveness data that were only collected by psychometric (or profile-based) instruments which measure the severity of the health problems but not the disutility or utility associated with the health outcomes. In such situations, CUA can be conducted only if there is a function available to convert the non-preference-based data into preference scores. Hence, such utility prediction functions are valuable in CUA. Recent years have seen an

Chapter 5
Predicting Preference-Based SF-6D$_{36}$ Index Scores from the SF-8 Health Survey

increasing number of studies developing functions to predict preference scores from profile-based quality-of-life instruments through the modeling approach (Brazier et al., 2002; Chuang and Kind, 2009; Sengupta et al., 2004; Ara and Brazier, 2009; Hanmer, 2009; Gray et al., 2006; Rowen et al., 2009; Cheung et al., 2008; Sullivan and Ghushchyan, 2006; Franks et al., 2004; Lawrence et al., 2004). Such prediction approach has been accepted by NICE as a valid method for generating utility scores for CUA (NICE, 2012).

The SF-8 is a recently developed tool within the class of SF health surveys, which are the most widely used health status measures in health outcomes research (Ware et al., 2001). It is derived from the SF-36 for the purposes of yielding comparable scores for the 8 health dimensions and 2 summary measures of the SF-36 with minimal respondent burden. While the SF-8 is substantially shorter than the SF-36, it covers a narrow range of SF-36 scores and less precise (Ware et al., 2001). Also, the SF-8 health survey is a profile-based instrument that can not be used to calculate QALYs. In contrast, methods have been available for deriving the preference-based SF-6D$_{36}$ score from the SF-36 and SF-12, both at the individual level and the group level (Ara and Brazier, 2009; Hanmer, 2009; Brazier and Roberts, 2002, 2004).

The aim of this study was to develop a function for generating the preference-based SF-6D$_{36}$ index scores from the SF-8. For this purpose, we tested seven different predicting models using data collected from a large-scale population health survey in which respondents completed.

5.2 Methods

5.2.1 SF-8

The SF-8 health survey is an 8-item health-related quality-of-life instrument. Each of the 8 items measures a different health dimension:

physical function (PF), role-physical(RP), bodily pain (BP), general health (GH), vitality (VT), social function (SF), mental health (MH), and role emotional (RE) (Ware et al., 2001). Each item uses a 5-point or 6-point Likert-type scale. The SF-8 raw item scores can be transformed into 8 dimension scores by assigning the mean SF-36 scale score from the 2,000 general US populations to each response category of the SF-8 measuring the same concept. Moreover, factor score coefficients are assigned to each item to generate two summary scores: the physical component summary (PCS) and the mental component summary (MCS) (Ware et al., 2001). Both dimension and the summary scores are scored with mean of 50 and standard deviation of 10 and higher scores indicating better health (Ware et al., 2001). The SF-8 has been well validated in various populations (Roberts et al., 2008; Bost et al., 2007; Lefante et al., 2005; Sugimoto et al., 2008) and the SF-36 from which the SF-8 was developed was also validated in Singapore (Thumboo et al., 2001).

5.2.2　SF-6D$_{36}$

Brazier et al. established a preference-based health measure from the SF-36 (Brazier et al., 2002). They used a selection of eleven SF-36 items to construct a six-attribute health classification system: physical function, role limitation, social function, pain, mental health, and vitality (Brazier et al., 2002). The SF-6D$_{36}$ system defines totally 18,000 health states. Using the standard gamble valuation technique, a representative sample of 611 members of the UK general population was interviewed to estimate the utility scores of the SF-6D$_{36}$ health states. The range of SF-6D$_{36}$ index score is from 0.296 to 1, where 0.296 corresponds to the worst health state and 1 corresponds to the best health state (Brazier et al., 2002). In our study, the SF-6D$_{36}$ scores were calculated using responses to the SF-36 questions.

5.2.3 Data

We developed the prediction equation using data from a previous cross-sectional survey investigating cardiovascular risk factors for the general population in Singapore (Wee et al., 2010). In this study, a total of 10,747 participants were interviewed face-to-face using a questionnaire consisted of the SF-8 health survey, the SF-36 health survey, and questions covering demographic characteristics, lifestyle factors, and health conditions. All participants were randomly selected from the Singapore general population, with a stratified sampling design to oversample the minority ethnic groups (Malays and Indians) (Wee et al., 2010).

5.2.4 Model construction

The overall aim of this study is to identify the "best" model for predicting the SF-6D$_{36}$ index scores based on the SF-8 data. Four groups of ordinary least-square (OLS) models with different independent variables were assessed for predicting the SF-6D$_{36}$ index scores. Model I used SF-8 raw item scores as predictors. The raw item score for each item ranges from 1 to 5 or 6, with 1 representing best level of health and 5 or 6 representing worst level. In this model, the 8 raw item scores were treated as continuous variables. Models II and Model III adopted the SF-8 dimension scores and summary scores (i.e. PCS and MCS) as independent variables, respectively. Model IV is similar to Model I in that the 8 raw items were the independent variables. However, the raw item scores were treated as categorical data in this case. Hence, dummy variables were generated for each item score. For instance, for the item measured on a 5-point scale for physical functioning, 4 dummy variables were generated.

All first-order two-way interactions of independent variables (including squared terms) were tested for Models I, Model II, and Model III.

Interactions were not tested for Model Ⅳ due to its similarity with Model Ⅰ. Therefore, we estimated a total of seven regression models: the main-effect models without interaction terms (Models Ⅰa, Model Ⅱa, Model Ⅲa, and Model Ⅳ) and the main-effect models with interaction terms (Models Ⅰb, Model Ⅱb, and Model Ⅲb). In our analyses, multicollinearity was examined but not resolved because the purpose of the modeling was to achieve good prediction rather than identifying predictors. The general form of the OLS models can be written as follows:

$$Y = \alpha + \beta_1 X_1 + \beta_2 X_2 + \varepsilon$$

where Y represents the SF-6D$_{36}$ index score; α is the regression intercept. X_1 indicates the SF-8 variables (main effect); and X_2 is the first-order interactions between the SF-8 variables. β_1 and β_2 are regression coefficients of the corresponding independent variables; and ε is the residual of the regression model. The stepwise variable elimination procedure was used for X_2 selection (Ara and Brazier, 2009).

5.2.5 Model estimation and evaluation

The predictive performance of the models was evaluated through a simple, one-round cross-validation approach. The study sample was randomly partitioned into two mutually exclusive subsets of equal size. One subset of data ("modeling" dataset) was used for model estimation while the other subset ("validation" dataset) was used for evaluating the prediction performance of the tested models. All models were assessed for predictive performance using a number of goodness-of-fit measures including adjusted R^2, root mean squared error (RMSE), mean absolute error (MAE), and percentage of prediction errors smaller than 0.05, 0.10, and the minimally important difference (MID) of SF-6D$_{36}$ scores (i.e. 0.042) (Walters and Brazier, 2005) in absolute magnitude. Distributional statistics (i.e. mean, standard deviation, maximum, and minimum) of the predicted SF-6D$_{36}$ index scores were also examined.

Model prediction was also assessed at the group level since the published SF-8 data were mostly in the form of mean values. For this purpose, a total number of 49 homogeneous subgroups of respondents were defined according to different demographics (i.e. age, gender, income, year of education, and house type) and chronic conditions (i.e. hypertension, diabetes, lung disease, pain, mental illness, cancer, and coronary heart disease) for both "modeling" and "validation" dataset. For each model tested, RMSE, MAE, and percentage of prediction errors less than the MID in absolute magnitude were calculated based on predicted and observed mean scores of those groups. In this analysis, the predicted group-level SF-6D$_{36}$ scores were calculated using the group mean SF-8 scores for Model Ⅰ, Model Ⅱ, and Model Ⅲ and the group proportion of each SF-8 items for Model Ⅳ.

We also assessed the interchangeability between the actual SF-6D$_{36}$ scores and predicted scores generated from all models using intraclass correlation coefficient (ICC). The ICC values range from 0 to 1, with larger values indicating higher degree of agreement (Fayers and Machin, 2005). ICC values of at least 0.7 and 0.9 are considered satisfactory for group comparison and individual comparison, respectively(Nunnally and Bernstein, 1994).

After the specifications of the aforementioned models were determined, model parameters were re-estimated using data from the entire sample (i.e., both "modeling" and "validation" datasets).

5.3 Results

A total of 7,529 respondents provided data for this study. The mean age of the sample was 50 years (range: 14—96), with female 52.6% of the total.

The distribution of SF-6D$_{36}$ index scores was skewed with mean and median being 0.796 (standard deviation: 0.124) and 0.845 (range: 0.319—1). The socio-demographic characteristics of the study sample and the distributions of the SF-8 and SF-6D$_{36}$ scores are summarized in Table 5.1.

5.3.1 Individual-level prediction

The main effects of all the independent variables in the 7 models were statistically significant when the models were tested with the "modeling" dataset. Table 5.2 shows the adjusted R^2 ranged from 55.9% to 62.1%, MAE ranged from 0.056 to 0.063, and RMSE ranged from 0.076 to 0.082; 42.5% to 51.5% of prediction errors was smaller than MID, 51.8%—59.2% of prediction errors was smaller than |0.05|, and 77.9%—84.3% of prediction errors was smaller than |0.10|. The mean predicted values were identical to the mean of the observed SF-6D$_{36}$ scores for all models; however, the standard deviation and the maximum of the predicted scores (range: 0.899—0.933) were smaller than those of the observed scores (highest score = 1.0) while the minimal predicted scores (range: 0.200—0.509) were either higher or lower than the observed minimal score (i.e. 0.319) depending on the model specifications. Furthermore, the predicted scores generated from models with interaction terms and Model Ⅳ were all within the possible range of SF-6D$_{36}$ scores (0.296—1). Among them, the PCS, MCS scores with interaction terms (Model Ⅲb) covered 80.6% of the actual range of SF-6D$_{36}$ scores (0.319—1) in the dataset compared with 60.6%—75.5% for other models. Plotting the residuals, predicted and actual SF-6D$_{36}$ scores showed that Model IIIb (Figure 5.1) and all other models (data not shown) predicted lower scores at the higher end of the SF-6D$_{36}$ scale and scores with greater variance at the lower end of the scale. Model fit was similar across models for the "validation" dataset (Table 5.3).

The ICC values at individual level ranged from 0.730 to 0.775 for the

Chapter 5
Predicting Preference-Based SF-6D$_{36}$ Index Scores from the SF-8 Health Survey

"modeling" dataset and 0.717—0.766 for the "validation" dataset, respectively.

Table 5.1 Socio-demographic characteristics and health status of the study sample ($N=7,529$)

	Number(%)	SF-6D$_{36}$		PCS-8		MCS-8	
		Mean	SD^a	Mean	SD	Mean	SD
Full sample	7,529(100.0)	0.796	0.124	52.22	6.32	52.84	6.66
Age(year)							
<45	2,748(36.5)	0.811	0.120	53.73	5.20	52.62	6.68
45–64	3,742(49.7)	0.797	0.121	52.10	5.95	53.16	6.40
≥65	971(12.9)	0.752	0.136	48.38	8.54	52.17	7.52
Gender							
Female	3,960(52.6)	0.782	0.126	51.56	6.57	52.39	6.88
Male	3,569(47.4)	0.812	0.120	52.95	5.94	53.32	6.38
Ethnicity							
Chinese	5,481(72.8)	0.804	0.123	52.21	6.05	52.92	6.33
Indian	648(8.6)	0.772	0.138	50.56	7.42	52.02	7.58
Malay	1,400(18.6)	0.792	0.133	51.31	6.15	53.09	6.41
Education							
No	459(6.1)	0.736	0.137	47.50	9.05	51.23	7.98
1–3 years	264(3.5)	0.780	0.126	50.16	7.28	53.06	6.36
4–6 years	1,242(16.5)	0.791	0.122	51.39	6.43	52.88	6.60
7–10 years	2,688(35.7)	0.796	0.123	52.23	6.11	53.00	6.54
≥10 years	2,681(38.0)	0.810	0.120	53.51	5.29	52.90	6.58
Monthly income(S$)							
≤2,000	1,318(17.5)	0.761	0.133	50.31	7.34	51.71	7.76
2 001–4,000	1,468(19.5)	0.794	0.129	51.98	6.16	53.09	6.90
4 001–6,000	715(9.5)	0.789	0.126	52.45	5.66	52.40	7.06
6 001–10,000	550(7.3)	0.802	0.114	53.34	4.93	53.05	6.32
>10000	324(4.3)	0.827	0.110	53.89	4.60	53.61	6.25
House type							
1 or 2 rooms	151(2.0)	0.766	0.138	49.88	8.33	51.16	7.96
3 rooms	1,182(15.7)	0.790	0.126	51.64	6.93	52.57	6.75
4 rooms	2,756(36.6)	0.797	0.123	52.12	6.18	52.78	6.54
5 rooms	2,281(30.3)	0.795	0.124	52.49	6.21	52.79	6.88
Condo	625(8.3)	0.807	0.118	52.82	5.66	53.61	6.08
Landed	520(6.9)	0.810	0.126	52.90	5.68	53.41	6.34
Chronic conditions							
Hypertension	1,386(18.4)	0.762	0.131	49.47	7.55	52.21	7.18
Diabetes	647(8.6)	0.746	0.138	48.51	8.14	51.42	7.79
Coronary heart disease	399(5.3)	0.786	0.123	51.48	6.82	52.56	6.82
Lung disease	324(4.3)	0.777	0.130	51.30	6.60	52.31	7.12
Pain	1,363(18.1)	0.789	0.125	51.84	6.51	53.00	6.59
Mental illness	68(0.9)	0.796	0.125	51.51	7.33	52.30	7.22
Cancer	67(0.9)	0.787	0.130	51.04	6.92	52.36	6.71
Stroke	68(0.9)	0.676	0.148	41.42	11.27	47.59	12.42

SD: standard deviation; PCS-8: physical component summary of SF-8; MCS-8: mental component summary of SF-8

Measuring Health-State Utilities for Cost-Utility Analysis
测量健康效用以用于成本效用分析

Table 5.2 Goodness of fit of the tested OLS models in the modeling dataset

		Actual	Model Ⅰa	Model Ⅰb	Model Ⅱa	Model Ⅱb	Model Ⅲa	Model Ⅲb	Model Ⅳ
Individuals Level ($N=3,765$)	Mean	0.796	0.796	0.796	0.796	0.796	0.796	0.796	0.796
	SD	0.124	0.095	0.098	0.093	0.097	0.093	0.095	0.097
	Min	0.319	0.246	0.502	0.210	0.509	0.200	0.384	0.408
	Max	1.000	0.905	0.926	0.899	0.922	0.911	0.933	0.922
	Adj R^2		0.584	0.620	0.566	0.613	0.559	0.580	0.621
	MSE		0.006	0.006	0.007	0.006	0.007	0.006	0.006
	MAE		0.060	0.056	0.062	0.057	0.063	0.061	0.056
	RMSE		0.080	0.077	0.082	0.077	0.082	0.080	0.076
	<|0.10|*		79.3%	83.6%	77.9%	84.1%	78.2%	81.4%	84.3%
	<|0.05|*		53.4%	56.2%	51.8%	55.3%	52.2%	52.3%	59.2%
	<MID*		45.7%	50.3%	43.9%	48.8%	42.5%	45.0%	51.5%
Group level ($N=49$)	Mean	0.774	0.779	0.780	0.779	0.780	0.779	0.780	0.782
	SD	0.134	0.108	0.104	0.103	0.107	0.103	0.105	0.108
	Min	0.403	0.268	0.558	0.227	0.547	0.212	0.390	0.427
	Max	0.996	0.901	0.919	0.896	0.920	0.910	0.930	0.922
	ME		0.0051	0.0058	0.0051	0.0058	0.0049	0.0060	0.0079
	MAE		0.0077	0.0075	0.0076	0.0076	0.0076	0.0079	0.0091
	RMSE		0.0112	0.0108	0.0111	0.0105	0.0117	0.0119	0.0121
	<MID*		100%	100%	100%	99%	100%	100%	100%

Model Ⅰa: SF-8 raw item scores without interaction; Model Ⅰb: SF-8 raw item scores with interaction; Model Ⅱa: SF-8 dimension scores without interaction; Model Ⅱb: SF-8 dimension scores with interaction; Model Ⅲa: SF-8 PCS MCS scores without interaction; Model Ⅲb: SF-8 PCS MCS scores with interaction; Model Ⅳ: SF-8 raw item score model (treated as categorical data)

* Percentage of cases for whom the difference between actual and predicted scores was less than 0.10, 0.05, or MID(0.042)

OLS: ordinary least-square; SD: standard deviation; MSE: mean square error; MAE: mean absolute error; RMSE: root mean square error; MID: minimal important difference; ME: mean error

Table 5.3 Goodness of fit of the tested OLS models in the validation dataset

		Actual	Model Ⅰa	Model Ⅰb	Model Ⅱa	Model Ⅱb	Model Ⅲa	Model Ⅲb	Model Ⅳ
Individuals Level ($N=3,764$)	Mean	0.796	0.794	0.794	0.796	0.796	0.796	0.796	0.794
	SD	0.124	0.099	0.099	0.098	0.099	0.097	0.097	0.099
	Min	0.370	0.220	0.475	0.184	0.494	0.181	0.384	0.409
	Max	1.000	0.905	0.926	0.899	0.922	0.911	0.933	0.922
	MSE		0.006	0.006	0.007	0.006	0.007	0.006	0.006
	MAE		0.061	0.056	0.062	0.057	0.063	0.063	0.058
	RMSE		0.082	0.077	0.082	0.078	0.084	0.081	0.076

(To be continued)

Chapter 5
Predicting Preference-Based SF-6D$_{36}$ Index Scores from the SF-8 Health Survey

(Continued)

		Actual	Model Ⅰa	Model Ⅰb	Model Ⅱa	Model Ⅱb	Model Ⅲa	Model Ⅲb	Model Ⅳ
Individuals Level ($N=3,764$)	<|0.10|*		79.2%	83.5%	77.4%	83.6%	78.2%	81.3%	84.0%
	<|0.05|*		53.2%	56.1%	52.3%	54.8%	52.3%	51.9%	59.2%
	<MID*		46.6%	49.8%	45.4%	48.6%	43.4%	45.5%	51.3%
Group level ($N=49$)	Mean	0.784	0.781	0.783	0.780	0.782	0.780	0.781	0.785
	SD	0.138	0.111	0.110	0.110	0.111	0.109	0.106	0.112
	Min	0.401	0.265	0.539	0.224	0.543	0.210	0.391	0.423
	Max	0.998	0.902	0.921	0.897	0.921	0.911	0.933	0.922
	ME		−0.0034	−0.0010	−0.0041	0.0014	−0.0042	−0.0020	0.0009
	MAE		0.0075	0.0072	0.0080	0.0070	0.0075	0.0061	0.0073
	RMSE		0.0111	0.0099	0.0118	0.0097	0.0097	0.0091	0.0100
	<MID*		100%	100%	100%	100%	100%	100%	100%

Model Ⅰa: SF-8 raw item scores without interaction; Model Ⅰb: SF-8 raw item scores with interaction; Model Ⅱa: SF-8 dimension scores without interaction; Model Ⅱb: SF-8 dimension scores with interaction; Model Ⅲa: SF-8 PCS MCS scores without interaction; Model Ⅲb: SF-8 PCS MCS scores with interaction; Model Ⅳ: SF-8 raw item score model (treated as categorical data)

* Percentage of cases for whom the difference between actual and predicted scores was less than 0.10, 0.05, or MID(0.042)

OLS: ordinary least-square; SD: standard deviation; MSE: mean square error; MAE: mean absolute error; RMSE: root mean square error; MID: minimal important difference; ME: mean error

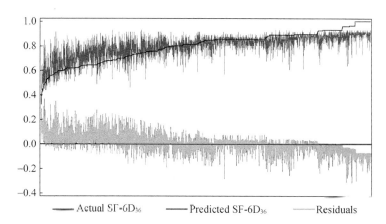

Figure 5.1 Residuals and SF-6D$_{36}$ scores predicted by Model Ⅲb (PCS, MCS, PCS * MCS) for the modeling dataset ($N=3,765$)

Observations are ordered from low to high according to the actual SF-6D$_{36}$ scores. The Y axis illustrates the magnitude of actual, predicted scores and residuals. The X axis shows different observations from low to high according to the actual SF-6D scores.

5.3.2 Group-level prediction

In general, all 7 models predicted similar-to-actual mean SF-$6D_{36}$ scores for 49 subgroups differing in demographics or health status. For each model, almost 100% proportion of the differences between observed and predicted means scores was smaller than the MID of SF-$6D_{36}$ (Table 5.2). The MAE and RMSE calculated based on these mean scores ranged from 0.0075 to 0.0091 and 0.0105 to 0.0121, respectively. Scatter plots (Figure 5.2) revealed that Model IIIb predicted slightly lower scores at the higher end of the SF-$6D_{36}$ scale for the "modeling" dataset. When the estimated models were applied to the "validation" dataset, similar goodness-of-fit results were observed (Table 5.3).

The ICC values at group level were 0.959—0.968 for "modeling" dataset and 0.949—0.954 for "validation" dataset, respectively.

Overall, for predicting both individual scores and group mean scores, the tested models had similar performance. However, the prediction performance at the group level was better than that at the individual level. The parameters of the 7 models estimated using the entire dataset were displayed in Table 5.4.

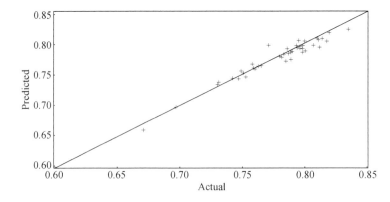

Figure 5.2 Scatter plot of actual and predicted mean SF-$6D_{36}$ scores for 49 subgroups of individuals based on the mean SF-8 PCS and MCS scores of the subgroups and their interaction term (i.e. Model Ⅲb)

Chapter 5
Predicting Preference-Based SF-6D$_{36}$ Index Scores from the SF-8 Health Survey

Table 5.4 The parameters of the 7 OLS models estimated using the entire dataset ($N=7,529$)

	Model Ia	Model Ib		Model IIa	Model IIb		Model IIIa	Model IIIb		Model IV 2	3	4	5	6
PF	-0.0212	-0.0490	PFnbs	0.0026	-0.0028	PCS	0.0093	-0.0046	PF	-0.0272	-0.0436	-0.0497	-0.0405	-0.0944
RP	-0.0097	-0.0162	RPnbs	0.0013	-0.0060	MCS	0.0084	-0.0056	RP	-0.0246	-0.0283	-0.0302	-0.0889	-0.0200
BP	-0.0262	-0.0486	BPnbs	0.0041	-0.0069	PCS*MCS		0.0003	BP	-0.0402	-0.0483	-0.0659	-0.0984	
GH	-0.0064	-0.0076	GHnbs	0.0011	0.0013				GH	-0.0059	-0.0110	-0.0231	-0.0186	
VT	-0.0219	-0.0564	VTnbs	0.0025	-0.0142				VT	-0.0313	-0.0507	-0.0631	-0.0408	
SF	-0.0224	-0.0475	SFnbs	0.0022	-0.0027				SF	-0.0362	-0.0307	-0.0506	-0.0705	
RE	-0.0252	-0.0613	REnbs	0.0036	-0.0163				RE	-0.0455	-0.0606	-0.0592	-0.0344	
MH	-0.0266	-0.0432	MHnbs	0.0036	-0.0035				MH	-0.0276	-0.0444	-0.0679	-0.1213	
Constant	1.0652	1.2158		-0.2908	1.3683		-0.1316	0.5462		0.9223				
VT * MH				0.0082		VT * MH		0.0001						
SF * RE				0.0146		PF * SF		0.0001						
PF * PF				0.0067		RP * RP		0.0001						
BP * BP				0.0049		BP * BP		0.0001						
VT * VT				0.0045		VT * VT		0.0001						

Model Ia: SF-8 raw item scores without interaction; Model Ib: SF-8 raw item scores with interaction; Model IIa: SF-8 dimension scores without interaction; Model IIb: SF-8 dimension scores with interaction; Model IIIa: SF-8 PCS MCS scores without interaction; Model IIIb: SF-8 PCS MCS scores with interaction; Model IV: SF-8 raw item score model (treated as categorical data)

OLS: ordinary least-square; PF: physical functioning; RP: role-physical; BP: bodily pain; GH: general health; VT: vitality; SF: social functioning; RE: role emotional; MH: mental health.

PFnbs: physical functioning normalized score; RPnbs: role-physical normalized score; BPnbs: bodily pain normalized score; GHnbs: general health normalized score;

VTnbs: vitality normalized score; SFnbs: social functioning normalized score; REnbs: role emotional normalized score; MHnbs: mental health normalized score.

PCS: physical component summary score; MCS: mental component summary score.

The interaction terms presented in the table were all statistically significant

5.4 Discussion

In this study, we developed and tested functions for predicting the SF-$6D_{36}$ scores from the SF-8. With these functions available, cost-utility analysis can be conducted in situations where patients' health outcomes are only measured by the SF-8 without any preference-based health measures. To the best of our knowledge, there is no function for estimating utility index scores from the SF-8.

While the OLS models we tested can successfully predict SF-$6D_{36}$ scores, our models do not fit the data as well as the models developed by Ara and Brazier(2009) for the SF-36 and Hanmer(2009) for the SF-12. The adjusted R^2 of the OLS functions we tested was 56%—58%, respectively, compared to the R^2 in those two studies ranged from 83% to 88%. Similarly, when modeling the individual-level data, approximately 50%—80% of predicted values were with an error of <0.05—0.10, respectively, in our study. In contrast, 77%—95% of predicted SF-$6D_{36}$ scores were with an error of <0.05 and <0.10, respectively, in Ara and Brazier's model. The relatively higher goodness of fit of their models could be due to that the SF-$6D_{36}$ was derived from the SF-36 or SF-12 but not the SF-8.

In general, the OLS models performed well at the group level in predicting mean SF-$6D_{36}$ scores. In our study, the ICC values were all above the threshold for group comparison. The difference between predicted and observed SF-$6D_{36}$ mean scores is smaller than the MID of SF-$6D_{36}$ scores (i.e. 0.042) for almost all of the 49 subgroups (Table 5.2 and Table 5.3). In contrast, only 90% of subgroup mean scores were predicted with an error smaller than the MID in Ara and Brazier's study(2009). Hence, it seems that the functions we developed can be used to generate preference-based SF-$6D_{36}$ scores for groups of individuals whose health status are measured by the SF-8, if investigators need to perform post hoc cost-utility analysis. Although

Chapter 5
Predicting Preference-Based SF-6D$_{36}$ Index Scores from the SF-8 Health Survey

all functions we examined have similar performance in predicting SF-6D$_{36}$ scores, the function using the SF-8 PCS and MCS scores, and their interaction term (Model Ⅲb) could be more useful than other models in practice. First, the predicted scores cover most of the actual SF-6D$_{36}$ range. Second, in the literature, the SF-8 data are usually published in mean PCS, MCS, and/or dimension scores that can also be used to estimate PCS and MCS scores. Third, the function is parsimonious by using less number of parameters. Meanwhile, it should be noted that the Model Ⅲb and all other models with interaction terms predicted higher scores at the lower end of the SF-6D scale. Hence, using the model to predict low SF-6D scores is not recommended. It also should be noted that Model Ⅰ and Model Ⅳ, although modeled the same effect, showed different goodness-of-fit statistics. This is not surprising because Model Ⅳ has many more independent variables than Model Ⅰ.

On the other hand, the models we tested were not as satisfactory in making predictions at the individual level compared to making predictions at the group level. The difference between predicted and actual scores reached or exceeded the minimally important difference of SF-6D$_{36}$ scores (Table 5.2, Table 5.3) for a large proportion of the individuals in our study sample and great prediction errors existed in the lower end of the SF-6D$_{36}$ scale (Figure 5.1). Also, all predicted scores were with ICC values less than 0.9 indicating that they are not interchangeable with actual SF-6D$_{36}$ scores. Hence, using these models to predict SF-6D$_{36}$ scores at the level of individual subjects is not recommended.

Two technical issues related to our modeling strategies are worth discussion. First, we chose to use the OLS model to analyze our data. This decision was based on the fact that the OLS model was used in most studies mapping a profile-based measure onto a preference-based measure (Brazier et al., 2010). We noted that some investigators found the CLAD (Sullivan and Ghushchyan, 2006) and two-part (Li and Fu, 2009) models performed better than the OLS model for data with ceiling effects (i.e. a large proportion of individuals in the study sample being in full health). As only 4.95% of individuals in our study sample had a SF-6D$_{36}$ score of 1.0, we did not consider such models in our main analysis. Nevertheless, we subsequently modeled our data using the Tobit model, a two-part model (logistic plus OLS), the nonlinear spline model, and two neural networks models. None of these models outperformed the OLS model (data not shown but available on request). Second, the stepwise regression we used is a controversial method. However, it is less of a concern in the present study since our study was exploratory and our goal was to achieve the best model fit. Pervious mapping studies also used the stepwise selection method (Ara and Brazier, 2009). We subsequently applied forward, backward, least angle regression (LAR), and Lasso method to the model containing the main effects and all first-order interaction terms of the two SF-8 summary scores but the resultant model specifications did not give better predictions than Model Ⅲbs (data not shown but available on request). That more sophisticated methods did not produce better results suggested that the stepwise OLS model is sufficient for modeling our data.

Our study has some limitations that should be noted. First, the prediction functions we came up with are based on data from a sample of the general population in which the proportion of very ill individuals was low. As a result, the prediction accuracy of the functions may not be high for patient populations with poor health status. Similarly, our OLS prediction functions may not work well in very healthy general populations, as a much higher proportion of individuals in such populations should be in full health (i.e. utility score = 1.0). Second, the external validity of the functions is not evaluated as we do not have other datasets that contain both SF-8 and SF-6D$_{36}$ data from same respondents thus far. Without external validations, the usefulness of the resultant functions cannot be confirmed. Third, we were not able to assess the validity of the predicted scores by comparing those values

Chapter 5
Predicting Preference-Based SF-6D$_{36}$ Index Scores from the SF-8 Health Survey

with directly measured utility scores. Actually, this is a limitation of all mapping studies, that is, validity is only assessed by model fit. The strategy of deriving utility scores through a mapping function would benefit from comparison with utility scores for the health states of interest measured using direct techniques such as standard gamble or time trade-off. Fourth, the SF-6D$_{36}$ index scores were calculated using UK algorithm since the Singapore algorithm is absent. It is possible that the results and conclusions would be significantly different if using local algorithm. Hence, future studies are warranted to compare our results with results based on local algorithm if it is developed.

In conclusion, our study developed and compared prediction functions to generate preference-based SF-6D$_{36}$ index scores from the SF-8 health survey, the first of its kind. The functions tested in the present study make cost-utility analyses possible with the SF-8 data. Future research is needed to further evaluate the performance and external validity of the recommended prediction functions.

Chapter 6

Preference-Based SF-6D Scores Derived from the SF-36 and SF-12 Have Different Discriminative Power in a Population Health Survey

6.1 Introduction

The SF-6D (Brazier et al., 2002) is an instrument for describing and valuing individuals' health. It is designed for generating a preference-based index score suitable for cost-effectiveness analysis from the SF-36 (Ware et al., 1993). The SF-6D index score can also be estimated for individuals on the basis of their responses to the SF-12 (Brazier and Roberts, 2004) a profile-based instrument comprising 12 of the SF-36 items (Ware et al., 1996). The availability of multiple approaches to generating the SF-6D score raises the issue of comparability between its 2 variants, namely, the SF-$6D_{36}$ and SF-$6D_{12}$. Indeed, the SF-$6D_{36}$ score was found to be lower than the SF-$6D_{12}$ score in both patient and general population samples (Pickard et al., 2005; Hanmer, 2009), although they demonstrated similar responsiveness to change in a study of multiple patient groups (Brazier and Roberts, 2004). Evidence on sensitivity to differences in the cross-sectional comparison of different groups (also referred to as discriminative power) (Streiner and Norman, 1995) was documented for both SF-$6D_{36}$ (Petrou and Hockley, 2005) and SF-$6D_{12}$ (Cunillera et al., 2010); however, it is not known whether the 2 SF-6D scores have similar discriminative power.

Chapter 6
Preference-Based SF-6D Scores Derived from the SF-36 and SF-12 Have Different Discriminative Power in a Population Health Survey

The purpose of the present study was to compare the ability of the SF-$6D_{12}$ and SF-$6D_{36}$ to discriminate between different levels of health status in population health surveys. We also included 3 commonly used preference-based heath indices, namely, the EQ-5D-3L (Dolan, 1996), HUI2 (Torrance et al., 1996), and HUI3 (Feeny et al., 2002), in this study as external comparators.

6.2 Methods

6.2.1 Data source

We used data from the 2005 to 2006 National Health Measurement Study (NHMS), a cross-sectional health survey of the noninstitutionalized US population (Fryback et al., 2007). The NHMS surveyed 4,334 individuals using a random-digit dialed telephone interview method. A stratified sampling design was used to oversample blacks and older persons. Respondents (n = 3,522) with complete data for the EQ-5D-3L, HUI2, HUI3, SF-36, and the profile of chronic medical conditions were included in the present study. The presence or absence of each of 11 conditions (i.e, coronary heart disease, stroke, diabetes, arthritis, eye disease, sleep disorder, respiratory disease, depression, ulcer, thyroid disease, and back pain) was assessed from respondents using the question "Have you ever been told by a doctor or other health professional that you had ...?"

6.2.2 Instruments

The SF-36 (version 2.0), EQ-5D-3L, and HUI questionnaires were used to collect data for generating the SF-6D, EQ-5D-3L, HUI2, and HUI3 scores, respectively. Each of these preference-based instruments consists of

Measuring Health-State Utilities for Cost-Utility Analysis
测量健康效用以用于成本效用分析

2 components: a multiattribute classification system for describing an individual's health and a utility function for assigning each described health state a preference score. The classification systems define health using 5—8 different attributes or dimensions, each with 3—6 descriptors or levels. For all the instruments, their index scores reflect the health preferences of a general population and are measured on a scale anchored by 0 (corresponding to death) and 1.0 (corresponding to full health) (Brazier et al., 2002; Brazier and Roberts, 2004; Dolan, 1997; Torrance et al., 1996; Feeny et al., 2002). The main characteristics of the preference-based instruments are shown in Table 6.1. The 6-dimension classification systems of the SF-6D$_{36}$ and SF-6D$_{12}$ are identical in 3 dimensions, namely, role limitations, social functioning, and vitality; however, physical functioning (6 levels vs. 3 levels), bodily pain (6 levels vs. 5 levels), and mental health (depression and nervousness vs. depression only) are defined with more levels or aspects in SF-6D$_{36}$ than in SF-6D$_{12}$. These differences are because the SF-6D$_{36}$ and SF-6D$_{12}$ systems are based on 11 and 7 SF-12/36 items, respectively. Accordingly, the SF-6D$_{36}$ and SF-6D$_{12}$ define 18,000 and 7,500 unique health states, respectively. As preference values for the SF-6D health states were not available from the US population, those estimated from the general UK population were used in this study (Brazier et al., 2002; Brazier and Roberts, 2004).

Table 6.1 Characteristics of the preference-based instruments

	SF-6D$_{36}$	SF-6D$_{12}$	EQ-5D-3L	HUI2	HUI3
Classification system					
Dimension or attribute (no. levels)	PF(6)	PF(3)	Mobility(3)	Mobility(5)	Ambulation(6)
	MH(5)	MH(5)	AD(3)	Emotion(5)	Emotion(5)
	BP(6)	BP(5)	PD(3)	Pain(5)	Pain(5)
	SF(5)	SF(5)	UA(3)	Cognition(4)	Cognition(6)
	RL(4)	RL(4)	Self-care(3)	Self-care(4)	Dexterity(6)
	Vitality(5)	Vitality(5)		Sensation(4)	Hearing(6)
					Speech(5)
					Vision(6)

(To be continued)

Chapter 6
Preference-Based SF-6D Scores Derived from the SF-36 and SF-12 Have Different Discriminative Power in a Population Health Survey

(Continued)

	SF-6D$_{36}$	SF-6D$_{12}$	EQ-5D-3L	HUI2	HUI3
No. health states defined	18,000	7,500	243	24,000	972,000
Preference score Range	0.296–1.0	0.345–1.0	−0.11–1.0	−0.03–1.0	−0.36–1.0
Elicitation technique	Standard gamble	Standard gamble	Time trade-off	Standard gamble	Standard gamble
Country where the health preferences are from	UK	UK	US	Canada	Canada

AD: anxiety/depression; BP: bodily pain; PF: physical functioning; MH: mental health; SF: social functioning; RL: role limitations; PD: pain/discomfort; UA: usual activities

6.2.3 Data analysis

Discriminative power was assessed according to the instruments' relative efficiency in distinguishing respondents with and without a chronic condition. Relative efficiency of 2 instruments was defined as the ratio of F statistics in the analysis of variance (ANOVA) tests of the difference in their index scores between the 2 comparison groups (Fayers and Machin, 2000). As a higher F-statistic value is more likely to lead to statistical significance, the instrument with a higher F statistic would be considered more efficient or discriminative. In the present study, we used the instrument with the largest F statistic as the reference (relative efficiency = 1) to calculate the relative efficiency values of all other instruments (range, 0—1). Relative efficiency of the study instruments was assessed for each of 11 chronic conditions.

As the discriminative power of a preference-based instrument is partially dependent on its health state classification system, we assessed the classification efficiency of the dimension scales used by each instrument using the Shannon index (H') (Shannon, 1948). H' is defined as:

$$H' = -\sum_{i=1}^{L} p_i \log_2 p_i$$

Where L is the number of descriptive levels of a dimension scale and p_i is the proportion of respondents who endorse the ith level ($i = 1...L$). Larger H' values indicate higher classification efficiency. In the case of an even (rectangular) distribution, that is, individuals are evenly distributed among all levels, H' reaches its maximum that equals $\log_2 L$. Widely used as a measure of biodiversity, the Shannon index has also been used to assess health state classification systems (Janssen et al., 2007). As no guidelines were available for interpreting H', we calculated the 95% confidence intervals for H' using a bootstrap method (Efron and Tibshirani, 1993).

The discriminative power of the SF-6D$_{36}$ and SF-6D$_{12}$ was also compared in respondents who were on the ceiling of the EQ-5D-3L, HUI2, or HUI3 scale. These were respondents who reported full health with one of those instruments. We expected variation in health status among those respondents and hypothesized that the SF-6D is discriminative between those with and without chronic conditions.

All analyses were performed using SAS survey commands (Version 9.2) (e.g. surveymean and surveyfreq) to account for the complex sampling design (i.e. combination of multi-stage stratified sampling and post-stratification) of NHMS.

6.3 Results

The characteristics of the study sample and the population it represented are summarized in Table 6.2. After adjusting for the complex sampling design, the mean age of the respondents was 53.9 years, with 52.3% being women; 71.9% of the respondents reported one or more chronic conditions, with the 3 most prevalent conditions being arthritis (39.4%), eye disease (28.2%), and back pain (18.3%). The proportion of respondents reporting full health on the SF-6D$_{36}$ and SF-6D$_{12}$ was 4.3% and 8.6%, respectively,

Chapter 6
Preference-Based SF-6D Scores Derived from the SF-36 and SF-12 Have Different Discriminative Power in a Population Health Survey

and ranged from 13.6% (HUI2) to 44.3% (EQ-5D-3L) for other health index scores; floor effects (i.e. reporting of the worst possible health with an instrument) were observed only for the SF-6D$_{12}$ (0.2%) and HUI3 (0.1%).

Table 6.2 Demographic characteristics of the study sample

Variable	Level	%(N), unweighted	%, weighted
Gender	Male	43.1(1,518)	47.4
	Female	56.9(2,004)	52.3
Age	35-44 years	17.3(608)	32.2
	45-64 years	40.3(1,420)	44.2
	65-89 years	42.4(1,494)	23.6
Race	White	66.6(2,346)	82.3
	Black	28.7(1,012)	10.7
	Other	4.3(150)	7.0
	(Missing)	0.4(14)	0.1
Annual household income	< $20,000	19.3(678)	9.7
	$20,000-34,999	18.1(637)	14.1
	$35,000-74,999	31.3(1,104)	35.2
	$75,000+	23.5(829)	35.7
	(Missing)	7.8(274)	5.3
Education level	< High school	11.1(391)	7.5
	High school	30.4(1,058)	28.0
	Some post-high school	22.3(784)	22.1
	College or higher degree	36.0(1,268)	42.1
	(Missing)	0.6(21)	0.4
Work status	Working	54.5(1,921)	68.9
	Not working	45.3(1,597)	31.1
	Refused	0.1(2)	0.0
	(Missing)	0.1(2)	0.0

The mean SF-6D$_{36}$ score was lower than the mean SF-6D$_{12}$ score for the entire sample (0.792 and 0.821, respectively) and for respondents with and without a chronic condition by approximately 0.03 points (Table 6.3, $P < 0.001$ for all comparisons).

Compared with the SF-6D$_{12}$, the SF-6D$_{36}$ exhibited higher relative efficiency for 8 of the 11 conditions (Figure 6.1). Compared with all other instruments, the SF-6D$_{36}$ had the highest relative efficiency in 5 chronic conditions (diabetes, sleep disorder, respiratory disease, thyroid disease, and back pain), followed by EQ-5D-3L in 3 conditions (stroke, arthritis, and

Measuring Health-State Utilities for Cost-Utility Analysis
测量健康效用以用于成本效用分析

Table 6.3 The SF-6D$_{36}$ and SF-6D$_{12}$ scores for respondents with and without a chronic condition

Chronic condition (N)	Respondents with the condition			Respondents without the condition		
	Mean SF-6D$_{36}$ score (SE)	Mean SF-6D$_{12}$ score (SE)	Difference*	Mean SF-6D$_{36}$ score (SE)	Mean SF-6D$_{12}$ score (SE)	Difference*
CHD(403)	0.719(0.012)	0.745(0.013)	0.026	0.799(0.004)	0.828(0.004)	0.029
Stroke(183)	0.711(0.026)	0.735(0.025)	0.024	0.795(0.003)	0.824(0.004)	0.029
Diabetes(621)	0.733(0.010)	0.762(0.011)	0.029	0.800(0.004)	0.829(0.004)	0.029
Arthritis(1,355)	0.731(0.006)	0.767(0.007)	0.036	0.819(0.004)	0.845(0.004)	0.026
Eye disease(969)	0.757(0.006)	0.790(0.007)	0.033	0.801(0.004)	0.829(0.004)	0.028
Sleep disorder(307)	0.680(0.014)	0.704(0.016)	0.024	0.802(0.003)	0.831(0.004)	0.029
Respiratory disease(555)	0.717(0.010)	0.744(0.011)	0.027	0.803(0.004)	0.832(0.004)	0.029
Depression(486)	0.691(0.011)	0.713(0.012)	0.022	0.810(0.003)	0.840(0.004)	0.030
Ulcer(421)	0.716(0.012)	0.742(0.012)	0.026	0.801(0.003)	0.830(0.004)	0.029
Thyroid(424)	0.752(0.009)	0.786(0.011)	0.034	0.797(0.004)	0.826(0.004)	0.029
Back pain(636)	0.684(0.008)	0.717(0.009)	0.033	0.815(0.003)	0.842(0.004)	0.027
Any of the above conditions(2,553)	0.790(0.005)	0.758(0.004)	0.032	0.877(0.005)	0.853(0.005)	0.024

* $P<0.001$ for all conditions; CHD: coronary heart disease; N: number of respondents observed in the study sample; SE: standard error

Chapter 6
Preference-Based SF-6D Scores Derived from the SF-36 and SF-12 Have Different Discriminative Power in a Population Health Survey

eye disorder), HUI2 in 2 conditions (coronary heart disease and ulcer), and SF-6D$_{12}$ in 1 condition (depression). Among the SF-6D$_{12}$, EQ-5D-3L, HUI2, and HUI3, none of the instruments had better F-statistic values than all the others (Figure 6.1).

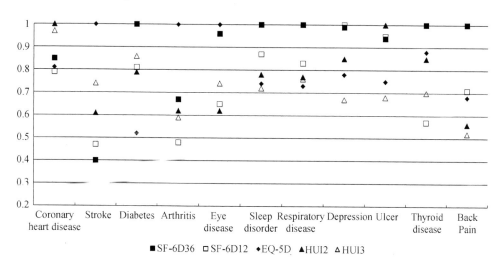

Figure 6.1 Relative efficiency of the SF-6D$_{36}$, SF-6D$_{12}$, EQ-5D-3L, HUI2, and HUI3 index scores in discriminating between respondents with and without a chronic condition

The SF-6D$_{36}$ had higher H' values than the SF-6D$_{12}$ in the 3 dimensions where their descriptive levels are different (Table 6.4). For example, the H' value (95% confidence interval) for the dimension of physical functioning was 1.73(1.67—1.79) and 0.78(0.72—0.85) in the SF-6D$_{36}$ and SF-6D$_{12}$, respectively. The SF-6D$_{36}$ also had higher H' values than all other instruments for dimensions assessing similar aspects of health. H' values for the similar dimensions of the SF-6D$_{12}$, EQ-5D-3L, HUI2, and HUI3 were similar (Table 6.4).

The SF-6D$_{36}$ exhibited higher relative efficiency in discriminating between respondents with and without chronic conditions than the SF-6D$_{12}$ in respondents on the ceiling of the EQ-5D-3L, HUI2, or HUI3 scale (Table 6.5). Moreover, using 0.041 as the minimally important difference (Walters and Brazier, 2005), the SF-6D$_{36}$ indicated that the impact of chronic conditions

Measuring Health-State Utilities for Cost-Utility Analysis
测量健康效用以用于成本效用分析

Table 6.4 Classification efficiency of the SF–6D$_{36}$, SF–6D$_{12}$, EQ–5D–3L, HUI2, and HUI3 systems measured by Shannon's Indices

SF–6D$_{36}$		SF–6D$_{12}$		EQ–5D–3L		HUI2		HUI3	
Dimension	H'(95%CI)	Dimension	H'(95%CI)	Dimension	H'(95%CI)	Dimension	H'(95%CI)	Dimension	H'(95%CI)
PF	1.73(1.67–1.79)	PF	0.78(0.72–0.85)	Mobility	0.73(0.67–0.78)	Mobility	0.95(0.90–1.01)	Ambulation	0.62(0.55–0.69)
MH	1.70(1.65–1.74)	MH	1.39(1.32–1.45)	AD	0.82(0.77–0.88)	Emotion	1.15(1.09–1.21)	Emotion	1.06(0.99–1.13)
BP	2.16(2.12–2.21)	BP	1.56(1.50–1.62)	PD	1.16(1.12–1.19)	Pain	1.69(1.64–1.74)	Pain	1.83(1.78–1.90)
SF	1.40(1.33–1.48)	SF	1.40(1.33–1.48)	UA	0.75(0.69–0.80)	Cognition	1.09(1.04–1.13)	Cognition	1.51(1.45–1.59)
RL	1.65(1.60–1.70)	RL	1.65(1.60–1.70)	Self-care	0.24(0.20–0.28)	Self-care	0.18(0.13–0.23)	Dexterity	0.23(0.19–0.29)
Vitality	1.79(1.73–1.86)	Vitality	1.79(1.73–1.86)			Sensation	1.21(1.16–1.26)	Hearing	0.30(0.25–0.35)
								Speech	0.13(0.10–0.18)
								Vision	1.13(1.08–1.18)

PF: physical functioning; MH: mental health; BP: bodily pain; SF: social functioning; RL: role limitation; AD: anxiety/depression; PD: pain/discomfort; UA: usual activities. CI: confidence interval

Chapter 6
Preference-Based SF-6D Scores Derived from the SF-36 and SF-12 Have Different Discriminative Power in a Population Health Survey

on the health of respondents who reported full health with each of the 3 instruments was not trivial; in contrast, the SF-6D$_{12}$ failed to capture this impact for respondents who were on the ceiling of the EQ-5D-3L or HUI3 scale (Table 6.5).

Table 6.5 The SF-6D$_{36}$ and SF-6D$_{12}$ scores for respondents with and without chronic conditions among those who were on the ceiling of the EQ-5D-3L, HUI2, or HUI3 scale

Instrument	Presence of any chronic conditions	SF-6D$_{36}$		SF-6D$_{12}$		Relative efficiency*
		Mean(SD)	Difference	Mean(SD)	Difference	
EQ-5D-3L	Yes	0.891(0.083)	0.042 §	0.901(0.079)	0.033	0.68
	No	0.849(0.092)		0.877(0.093)		
HUI2	Yes	0.908(0.087)	0.055 §	0.925(0.082)	0.043 §	0.51
	No	0.853(0.102)		0.882(0.101)		
HUI3	Yes	0.899(0.094)	0.053 §	0.913(0.093)	0.036 †	0.47
	No	0.846(0.109)		0.877(0.106)		

SD: standard deviation
* Calculated as F-statistic of SF-6D$_{12}$ divided by F-statistic of SF-6D$_{36}$; § Difference larger than minimally important difference of 0.041; † $P<0.001$, for all the rest: $P<0.0001$.

6.4 Discussion

In this study, we found that the SF-6D$_{36}$ is more efficient than the SF-6D$_{12}$ and 3 other commonly used preference-based health indices in discriminating between individuals in differing health conditions. Thus, our study explains why the SF-6D was more discriminative than the EQ-5D-3L in Petrou and Hockley's study(2005) but not so in Cunillera et al's(2010) or Bharmal and Thomas's study(2006). The SF-6D score was derived from the SF-36 in Petrou and Hockley's study but from the SF-12 in the other 2 studies. It is not surprising that the SF-6D$_{36}$ is more discriminative than the SF-6D$_{12}$ because the SF-6D$_{36}$ describes health in greater detail than the SF-6D$_{12}$; however, previously, there was no evidence on this. Hence, our study makes a strong case for using the SF-6D derived from the SF-36 in population health surveys where a preference-based heath index is needed.

Consistent with the finding from the present study, the SF-6D$_{36}$ index score was lower than the SF-6D$_{12}$ index score in all age groups by as much as 0.042 in a previous population health survey (Hanmer, 2009). This difference may be due to the recommended utility functions assigning the score of 1.0 to both the SF-6D$_{36}$-defined and SF-6D$_{12}$-defined full health, although the former is better than the latter. Physical functioning in the SF-6D$_{36}$ and SF-6D$_{12}$ full health is defined as no limitations in "vigorous activities" and "moderate activities," respectively. Given this finding, comparison of absolute SF-6D scores derived from the SF-12 and SF-36 should be conducted with caution. The existence of this systematic difference, however, does not necessarily mean that SF-6D$_{12}$ and SF-6D$_{36}$ can not lead to similar results when they are used to quantify between group differences or within-group changes over time. In the present study, the magnitude of difference in health between respondents with and without a condition estimated by the SF-6D$_{36}$ and SF-6D$_{12}$ was very similar for all 11 conditions. For example, respondents with and without arthritis differed by 0.088 and 0.078 according to the SF-6D$_{36}$ and SF-6D$_{12}$, respectively (Table 6.3). Also, health changes occurring in patient groups assessed by these 2 SF-6D scores were found to be similar for a number of conditions (Brazier and Roberts, 2004; Pickard et al., 2005).

Our finding that the SF-6D$_{36}$ was more discriminative than the EQ-5D-3L is consistent with the finding from a previous study comparing these 2 instruments in a population health survey in England (Petrou and Hockley, 2005). Similar to our studies, previous studies also found that the SF-6D$_{12}$, EQ-5D-3L, HUI2, and HUI3 have similar measurement properties (Janssen et al., 2007; Bharmal et al., 2006; Luo et al., 2009). The better performance of SF-6D$_{36}$ than other instruments is likely due to its classification system. On the basis of the results from this study, it seems that the components of the SF-6D$_{36}$ are more optimal, as evaluated in a community sample. A fundamental difference between the SF-6D$_{36}$ and other instruments is the use

Chapter 6
Preference-Based SF-6D Scores Derived from the SF-36 and SF-12 Have Different Discriminative Power in a Population Health Survey

of descriptors for positive aspects of health (i.e. "a lot of energy" and "vigorous activities") in the SF-6D$_{36}$ classification system. Those positive health descriptors should be the reason for the minimal ceiling effects of the SF-6D$_{36}$ and its ability to detect variation in health that is beyond the measurement scope of other instruments.

On the basis of a general population sample, our findings may not be generalized to patient populations. A number of studies compared the discriminative power of the SF-6D, EQ-5D-3L, HUI2, and/or HUI3 in patient populations and their findings varied depending on the (severity of) conditions investigated (Zhao et al., 2010; Hatoum et al., 2004; Marra et al., 2005; McTaggart-Cowan et al., 2008; Longworth et al., 2003; Boonen et al., 2007; Hawthorne et al., 2001; Lamers et al., 2006; Kontodimopoulos, 2010). For example, the SF-6D$_{36}$ was found to be more efficient than the EQ-5D-3L in patients with chronic prostatitis (Zhao et al., 2010) but less discriminative than the EQ-5D-3L and HUI3 in patients with rheumatoid arthritis (Marra et al., 2005).

One limitation of our study is deriving the SF-6D$_{12}$ from the SF-36. Respondents might have responded to the SF-12 questions differently if it had been administered as a stand-alone questionnaire. Nevertheless, Ware et al suggested that there was a high correlation between isolated SF-12 questions and the SF-12 items embedded in the SF-36 ($r = 0.999$) (Ware JE et al., 1998). Another limitation is that the study sample did not include individuals younger than 35 years of age. Thus, our findings may not be generalized to the very young adult population. Very young adults are generally either in full health or only in early stages of chronic conditions, if any.

In conclusion, the SF-36 provides a more discriminative preference-based health index than the SF-12. Findings from our study support the use of the SF-6D score derived from the SF-36 in population health surveys where a preference-based health index is needed.

Chapter 7

Conclusions

7.1 Major findings

I conducted several studies to address research questions on measuring HSUs. Major findings of these studies are as follows:

1) The utility of EQ-5D-5L health states is higher to the people in China than to Chinese Singaporeans.

2) The utility of mild EQ-5D-3L health states is higher to T2DM patients than to the general population and therefore the EQ-5D-3L values based on the general population's preferences could be insensitive to the benefits of and underestimate the effectiveness of health inventions for T2DM.

3) The values of EQ-5D-3L health states estimated using the TTO method in Singapore are lower and vary greater than those EQ-5D-3L values from other countries. Therefore, using EQ-5D-3L value sets from other countries would underestimate the health gain and cost-effectiveness of health interventions in Singapore.

4) The preference-based $SF-6D_{36}$ index score can be generated from the SF-8 health survey.

5) The SF-6D index score derived from the SF-36 is more efficient than that derived from the SF-12 as well as three other commonly used preference-based health indices (i.e. EQ-5D-3L, HUI2, and HUI3) in discriminating between individuals in different health conditions.

Chapter 7
Conclusions

7.2 Contributions

This book has contributed new knowledge to the understanding on HSU measurement for CUA. The main contributions are summarized as follows:

1) The difference in TTO values of EQ-5D-5L health states between the people in China and Chinese Singaporeans could lead to different CUA results if one population's preferences are used to the other population. Hence, the development of local EQ-5D-5L value sets is supported.

2) The utility of mild EQ-5D-3L health states are higher to T2DM patients than to the general population and therefore the EQ-5D-3L values based on the general population's preferences could be insensitive to the benefits of and underestimate the effectiveness of health inventions for T2DM. Hence, it might be worthwhile to determine the values of the EQ-5D-3L health states to patients with a certain condition and use patients' values to inform clinical decision making for the relevant disease.

3) The established EQ-5D-3L value set provides health services researchers a useful tool to appraise the cost-effectiveness of health technologies or interventions in Singapore.

4) The functions developed for predicting the preference-based SF-$6D_{36}$ index score from the psychometric instrument SF-8 enable the SF-8 data to be used in CUA.

5) The result that the SF-6D derived from the SF-36 is more discriminative than that derived from the SF-12 supports the usage of the SF-6D index score derived from the SF-36 whenever possible when a preference-based index is needed.

7.3 Future studies

The studies performed have also raised some new research questions worth exploring in future studies. These are:

1) Previously, researchers had to use the UK, US, or Japanese EQ-5D-3L value set to obtain utility scores in Singapore as there was no local EQ-5D-3L value set. Since we have established the local value set, future studies need to compare the Singapore EQ-5D-3L values with the values from other countries and to explore the impact of using other countries' values on CUAs in Singapore.

2) Future studies need to evaluate the performance of DCE in eliciting HSU values. Compared to prevailing valuation techniques (i.e. SG and TTO), the DCE is simpler and its values are less likely to be affected by factors other than preferences for health states. It is a promising tool in health-state valuation.

3) The EQ-5D-5L is a new version of the EQ-5D-3L, which has the same 5 domains as the EQ-5D-3L, but comprises 5 functional levels including no problems (level 1), slight problems (level 2), moderate problems (level 3), severe problems (level 4), and extreme problems (level 5). Currently, the EQ-5D-5L index score can be obtained by applying the indirect mapping method from the EQ-5D-3L to the EQ-5D-5L. Future studies need to develop EQ-5D-5L value sets based on directly measured EQ-5D-5L health states.

Chart Index

Table 1.1	Characteristics of the generic preference-based instruments	12
Table 2.1	Characteristics of participants	30
Table 2.2	Comparison of TTO values between the people in China and Chinese Singaporeans	32
Table 3.1	Characteristics of participants	42
Table 3.2	TTO values between T2DM patients and the general population	43
Table 4.1	Health states valued in the study	51
Table 4.2	Socio-demographic statistics of full sample and valuation sample compared with Singapore population	56
Table 4.3	Parameter estimates and goodness-of-fitness statistics at individual level using fixed effect (FE) and random effect (RE) regression	59
Table 4.4	Parameter estimates and goodness-of-fitness statistics at aggregated level using OLS regression	60
Table 5.1	Socio-demographic characteristics and health status of the study sample ($N = 7,529$)	75
Table 5.2	Goodness of fit of the tested OLS models in the modeling dataset	76
Table 5.3	Goodness of fit of the tested OLS models in the validation dataset	76

Table 5.4	The parameters of the 7 OLS models estimated using the entire dataset ($N=7,529$)	79
Table 6.1	Characteristics of the preference-based instruments	86
Table 6.2	Demographic characteristics of the study sample	89
Table 6.3	The SF-6D$_{36}$ and SF-6D$_{12}$ scores for respondents with and without a chronic condition	90
Table 6.4	Classification efficiency of the SF-6D$_{36}$, SF-6D$_{12}$, EQ-5D-3L, HUI2, and HUI3 systems measured by Shannon's Indices	92
Table 6.5	The SF-6D$_{36}$ and SF-6D$_{12}$ scores for respondents with and without chronic conditions among those who were on the ceiling of the EQ-5D-3L, HUI2, or HUI3 scale	93
Figure 1.1	SG for a health state considered as better than death	5
Figure 1.2	TTO for a health state considered as better than death	6
Figure 2.1	Mean TTO values for each of the 10 EQ-5D-5L health states between the people in China and Chinese Singaporeans	33
Figure 3.1	Mean TTO values for each of the 10 EQ-5D-5L health states between T2DM patients and the general population	44
Figure 4.1	Bland-Altman plots of actual and predicted scores based on OLS regression at aggregated level	62
Figure 5.1	Residuals and SF-6D$_{36}$ scores predicted by Model Ⅲb (PCS, MCS, PCS * MCS) for the modeling dataset ($N=3,765$)	77
Figure 5.2	Scatter plot of actual and predicted mean SF-6D$_{36}$ scores for 49 subgroups of individuals based on the mean SF-8 PCS and MCS scores of the subgroups and their interaction term (i.e. Model Ⅲb)	78
Figure 6.1	Relative efficiency of the SF-6D$_{36}$, SF-6D$_{12}$, EQ-5D-3L, HUI2, and HUI3 index scores in discriminating between respondents with and without a chronic condition	91

References

Abdin E, Subramanian M, Vaingankar J A, et al., 2013. Measuring health-related quality of life among adults in Singapore: population norms for the EQ-5D [J]. Quality of Life Research, 22:2983-2991.

Ara R, Brazier J, 2009. Predicting the short form-6D preference-based index using the eight mean short form-36 health dimension scores: estimating preference- based health-related utilities when patient level data are not available [J]. Value in Health, 12:346-353.

Attema A E, Edelaar-Peeters Y, Versteegh M M, et al., 2013. Time trade-off: one methodology, different methods [J]. The European Journal of Health Economics, 14(Suppl 1):53-64.

Badia X, Diaz Prieto A, Rue M, et al., 1996. Measuring health and health state preferences among critically ill patients [J]. Intensive Care Medicine, 22:1379-1384.

Badia X, Herdman M, Kind P, 1998. The influence of ill-health experience on the valuation of healths [J]. Pharmacoeconomics, 13:687-696.

Badia X, Roset M, Herdman M, et al., 2001. A comparison of United Kingdom and Spanish general population time trade-off values for EQ-5D health states [J]. Medical Decision Making, 21:7-16.

Bakker C, Rutten M, van Doorslaer E, et al., 1994. Feasibility of utility assessment by rating scale and standard gamble in patients with ankylosing spondylitis or fibromyalgia [J]. Journal of Rheumatology, 21:269-274.

Balaban D J, Sagi P C, Goldfarb N I, et al., 1986. Weights for scoring the quality of well-being instrument among rheumatoid arthritis: a comparison to general population weights [J]. Medical Care, 24:973-980.

BBC News, 2013. Survey finds 300m China believers [N/OL]. Available from:http://news.bbc.co.uk/2/hi/asia-pacific/6337627.stm.

Bharmal M, Thomas J 3rd, 2006. Comparing the EQ-5D and the SF-6D descriptive systems to assess their ceiling effects in the US general population [J]. Value in Health, 9:262-271.

Bland J M, Altman D G, 1986. Statistical method for assessing agreement between two methods of clinical measurement [J]. Lancet,1:307-310.

Bloom B S, 2004. Use of formal benefit/cost evaluations in health system decision making [J]. The American Journal of Managed Care, 10:329-335.

BMJ Group Blogs, 2013. BMJ Supportive & Palliative Care [EB/OL]. Available from: http://blogs.bmj.com/spcare/2012/04/17/one-can-die-but-cannot-fall-ill-a-survey-on-how-costs-may-affect-choice-of-therapy-in-singapore/.

Boonen A, van der Heijde D, Landewe R, et al., 2007. How do the EQ-5D, SF-6D and the well-being rating scale compare in patients with ankylosing spondylitis? [J]. Annals of Rheumatic Diseases, 66:771-777.

Bosch J L, Hammitt J K, Weinstein M C, et al., 1998. Estimating general population utilities using one binary-gamble question per respondent [J]. Medical Decision Making, 18:381-390.

Bost J E, Williams B A, Bottegal M T, et al., 2007. The 8-item Short-form Health Survey and the physical comfort composite score of the quality of recovery 40-item scale provide the most responsive assessments of pain, physical function, and mental function during the first 4 days after ambulatory knee surgery with regional anesthesia [J]. Anesthesia & Analgesia, 105:1693-1700.

Boyd N F, Sutherland H J, Heasman K Z, et al., 1990. Whose utilities for decision analysis? [J]. Medical Decision Making, 10:58-67.

Brazier J E, Roberts J, Deverill M D, 2002. The estimation of a preference-based measure of health from the SF-36 [J]. Journal of Health Economics,

21:271-292.

Brazier J E, Roberts J, 2004. The estimation of a preference-based measure of health from the SF-12 [J]. Medical Care, 42:851-859.

Brazier J, Akehurst R, Brennan A, et al., 2005. Should patients have a greater role in valuing health states? [J]. Applied Health Economics and Health Policy, 4:201-208.

Brazier J, Ratcliffe J, Salomon J, et al., 2007. Measuring and valuing health benefits for economic evaluation [M]. Oxford: Oxford University Press.

Brazier J E, Czoski-Murray C, Roberts J, et al., 2008. Estimation of a preference-based index from a condition specific measure: the Kind's Health Questionnaire [J]. Medical Decision Making, 28:113-126.

Brazier J E, Ratcliffe, J, 2008. The measurement and valuation of health for economic evaluation. In K. Heggenhougen, ed. International Encyclopaedia of Public Health [M]. San Diego: Academic Press.

Brazier J E, Yang Y, Tsuchiya A, et al., 2010. A review of studies mapping (or cross walking) non-preference based measures of health to generic preference-based measures [J]. The European Journal of Health Economics, 11: 215-225.

Breusch T, Pagan A, 1979. A Simple Test of Heteroskedasticity and Rrandom Coefficient Variation [J]. Econometrica, 47:1287-1294.

Brooks R, 1996. EuroQol: the current state of play [J]. Health Policy, 37: 53-72.

Buckingham K, Devlin N, 2006. A theoretical framework for TTO valuations of health [J]. Health Economics, 15:1149-1154.

Central Intelligence Agency, 2013. China. In: The World Fact Book [EB/OL]. Available from https://www.cia.gov/library/publications/the-world-factbook/geos/ch.html.

Chapman B P, Franks P, Duberstein P R, et al., 2009. Differences between individual and societal health state valuation: any link with personality? [J]. Medical Care, 10:902-907.

Measuring Health-State Utilities for Cost-Utility Analysis
测量健康效用以用于成本效用分析

Chong S A, Abdin E, Luo N, et al., 2012. Prevalence and impact of mental and physical comorbidity in the adult Singapore population [J]. Annals Academy of Medicine Singapore, 41: 105-114.

Cheung Y B, Tan L C, Lau P N, et al., 2008. Mapping the eight-item Parkinson's Disease Questionnaire (PDQ-8) to the EQ-5D utility index [J]. Quality of Life Research, 17: 1173-1181.

Chuang L H, Kind P, 2009. Converting the SF-12 into the EQ-5D: an empirical comparison of methodologies [J]. Pharmacoeconomics, 27: 491-505.

Clarke A E, Goldstein M K, Michelson D, et al., 1997. The effect of assessment method and respondent population on utilities elicited for Gaucher disease [J]. Quality of Life Research, 6: 169-184.

Cleemput L, 2010. A social preference valuation set for EQ-5D health states in Flanders, Belgium [J]. European Journal of Health Economics, 11: 205-213.

Coast J, Flynn T N, Natarajan J, et al., 2008. Valuing the ICECAP capability index for older people [J]. Social Science & Medicine, 67: 874-882.

Cunillera O, Tresserras R, Rajmil L, et al., 2010. Discriminative capacity of the EQ-5D, SF-6D, and SF-12 as measures of health status in population health survey [J]. Quality of Life Research, 19: 853-864.

Department of Statistic Singapore, 2013. Available from: http://www.singstat.gov.sg/publications/publications_and_papers/cop2010/census10_stat_release1.html.

Department of Statistic Singapore, 2013. Available from: http://www.singstat.gov.sg/publications/publications_and_papers/reference/sif2013.pdf.

De Wit G A, Busschbach J J, De Charro F T, 2000. Sensitivity and perspective in the valuation of health status: whose values count? [J]. Health Economics, 9: 109-126.

References

Devlin N J, Tsuchiya A, Buckingham K, et al., 2011. A uniform time trade off method for states better and worse than dead: feasibility study of the 'lead time' approach [J]. Health Economics, 20:348-361.

Dolders MGT, Zeegers MPA, Groot W, et al., 2006. A meta-analysis demonstrates no significant differences between patient and population preferences [J]. Journal of Clinical Epidemiology, 59:653-664.

Dolan P, Gudex C, Kind P, et al., 1996. Valuing health states: a comparison of methods [J]. Journal of Health Economics, 15:209-231.

Dolan P, 1997. Modeling valuations for EuroQol health states [J]. Medical Care, 35:1095-1108.

Dolan P (a), 1999. Whose preferences count? [J]. Medical Decision Making, 19:482-486.

Dolan P (b), 1999. Valuing health-related quality of life: Issues and controversies [J]. Pharmacoeconomics, 15:119-127.

Dobrez, D, Cella D, Pickard A S, et al., 2007. Estimation of patient preference-based utility weights from the functional assessment of cancer therapy-general [J]. Value in Health, 10:266-272.

Drummond M F, O'Brien B, Stoddart G L, et al., 2005. Methods for the Economic Evaluation of Health Care Programmes (3rd ed.) [M]. New York: Oxford University Press.

Edgar A, Salek S, Shickle D, et al., 1998. The ethical QALY: ethical issues in healthcare resource allocations. Haslemere: Euromed Communications.

Efron B, Tibshirani R J, 1993. An Introduction to the Bootstrap [M]. New York: Chapman & Hall.

Eleanor M P, Jean-Eric T, Xie F, et al., 2010. Analysis of health utility data when some subjects attain the upper bound of 1: are tobit and CLAD models appropriate? [J]. Value in Health, 13:487-494.

EuroQol Group, 2013. EQ-5D-5L User Guide [EB/OL]. Basic information on how to use the EQ-5D-5L instrument. Available from: http://www.euroqol.org/fileadmin/user _ upload/Documenten/PDF/Folders _ Flyers/

UserGuide_EQ-5D-5L.pdf.

Fayers P M, Machin D, 2005. Quality of life: Assessment, Analysis and Interpretation(3rd ed.) [M]. Chichester: John Wiley & Sons.

Feeny D, Furlong W, Boyle M, et al., 1995. Multi-attribute health status classification systems: health utilities index [J]. Pharmacoeconomics, 7: 490-502.

Feeny D H, Furlong W J, Torrance G W, et al., 2002. Multiattribute and single attribute utility functions for the health utilities index mark 3 system [J]. Medical Care, 40:113-128.

Feeny D, Eng K, 2005. A test of prospect theory [J]. International Journal of Technology Assessment in Health Care, 21:511-516.

Festinger L, 1957. A theory of cognitive dissonance [M]. Stanford: Stanford University Press.

Fitzpatrick R, Bowling A, Gibbons E, et al., 2006. A structured review of PROMs in relation of selected chronic conditions, perceptions of quality of care and carer impact [R]. Oxford: National Center for Health Outcomes Development.

Franks P, Lubetkin E I, Gold M R, et al., Mapping the SF-12 to the EuroQol EQ-5D index in a national US sample [J]. Medical Decision Making, 24:247-254.

Froberg D G, Kane R L, 1989. Methodology for measuring health state preferences Ⅱ: scaling methods [J]. Journal of Clinical Epidemiology, 42: 459-471.

Fryback D G, Dunham N C, Palta M, et al., 2007. US norms for six generic health-related quality-of-life indexes from the National Health Measurement study [J]. Medical Care, 45:1162-1170.

Fujiikee K, Mizuno Y, Hiratsuka Y, et al., 2011. Quality of life and cost-utility assessment after strabismus surgery in adults [J]. Japanese Journal of Ophthalmology, 55:268-276.

Gandjour A, 2010. Theoretical foundation of patient v. population preferences in calculating QALYs [J]. Medical Decision Making, 30: E57-63.

Gao F, Ng G Y, Cheung Y B, et al., 2009. The Singapore English and Chinese version of the EQ-5D achieved measurement equivalence in cancer patients [J]. Journal of Clinical Epidemiology, 62:206-213.

Golicki D, Jakubczyk M, Niewada M, et al., 2010. Valuation of EQ-5D health states in Poland: first TTO-based social value set in central and eastern Europe [J]. Value in Health, 13:289-297.

Gold M R, Siegel J E, Russell L B, et al., 1996. Cost-effectiveness in health and medicine [M]. Oxford: Oxford University Press.

Gray A M, Rivero-Arias O, Clarke P M, 2006. Estimating the association between SF-12 responses and EQ-5D utility values by response mapping [J]. Medical Decision Making, 26:18-29.

Green C, Brazier J, Deveril M, 2000. Valuing health-related quality of life. A review of health state valuation techniques [J]. Pharmacoeconomics, 17: 151-165.

Hanmer J, 2009. Predicting an SF-6D preference-based score using MCS and PCS scores from the SF-12 or SF-36 [J]. Value in Health, 12:958-966.

Hawthorne G, Richardson J, Day N A, 2001. A comparison of the Assessment of quality of life (AQol) with four other generic utility instruments [J]. Annals of Medicine, 33:358-370.

Hatoum H T, Brazier J E, Akhras K S, 2004. Comparison of the HUI3 with the SF-36 preference-based SF-6D in a clinical trial setting [J]. Value in Health, 7:602-609.

Hausman J, 1978. Specification tests in econometrics [J]. Econometrica, 46: 1251-1271.

Hicks J R, 1943. The four consumers' surpluses [J]. Review of Economic Studies, 11:31-41.

Hurst N P, Jobanputra P, Hunter M, et al., 1994. Validity of Euroqol: a generic health status instrument: in patients with rheumatoid arthritis.

Economic and Health Outcome Research Group [J]. British Journal of Rheumatology, 33:655-662.

Janssen M F, Birnie E, Bonsel G J, 2007. Evaluating the discriminatory power of EQ-5D, HUI2 and HUI3 in a US general population survey using Shannon's indices [J]. Quality of Life Research, 16:895-904.

Jelsma J, Hansen K, De Weerdt W, et al., 2003. How do Zimbabweans value health states? [J]. Population Health Metrics, 33:337-343.

Johannesson M, Jonsson B, Karlson G, 1996. Outcome measurement in economic evaluation [J]. Health Economics, 5:279-296.

Johnson J A, Luo N, Shaw J W, et al., 2005. Valuations of EQ-5D health states: are the United States and United Kingdom different? [J]. Medical Care, 43:221-228.

Johnson J A, Ohinmaa A, Murti B, et al., 2000. Comparison of Finnish and U.S.-based visual analog scale valuations of the EQ-5D measure [J]. Medical Decision Making, 20:281-289.

Kahneman D, Tversky A, 1982. The psychology of preference [J]. Scientific American, 246:160-173.

Kontodimopoulos N, Pappa E, Chadjiapostolou Z, et al., 2010. Comparing the sensitivity of EQ-5D, SF-6D and 15D utilities to the specific effect of diabetic complications [J]. The European Journal of Health Economics.

Kind P, Dolan P, 1995. The effect of past and present illness experience on the valuation of health states [J]. Medical Care, 33(Suppl 4):AS255-263.

Lamers L M, Bouwmans C A, van Straten A, et al., 2006. Comparison of EQ-5D and SF-6D utilities in mental health patients [J]. Health Economics, 15:1229-1236.

Lamers L M, McDonnell J, Stalmeier P F, et al., 2006. The Dutch tariff: results and arguments for an effective design for national EQ-5D valuation studies [J]. Health Economics, 15:1121-1132.

Lawrence W F, Fleishman J A, 2004. Predicting EuroQol EQ-5D preference scores from the SF-12 Health Survey in a nationally representative sample

[J]. Medical Decision Making, 24:160-169.

Lee Y K, Nam H S, Chuang L H, et al., 2009. South Korean time trade-off values for EQ-5D health states: modeling with observed values for 101 health states [J]. Value in Health, 12:1187-1193.

Lefante J J Jr, Harmon G N, Ashby K M, et al., 2005. Use of the SF-8 to assess health-related quality of life for a chronically ill, low-income population participating in the Central Louisiana Medication Access Program (CMAP) [J]. Quality of Life Research, 14:665-673.

Le Gales C, Buron C, Coster N, et al., 2002. Development of a preference-weighted health status classification system in France: the Health Utilities Index [J]. Health Care Manage Sci, 5:41-51.

Lenert L A, Treadwell J R, Schwartz C E, 1999. Association between health status utilities and implications for policy [J]. Medical Care, 37:479-489.

Llewellyn-Thomas H A, Sutherland H J, Tikshirani R, et al., 1982. The measurement of patients' values in medicine [J]. Medical Decision Making, 2:449-462.

Llewellyn-Thomas H, Sutherland H J, Tibshirani R, et al., 1984. Describing health states: methodologic issues in obtaining values for health states [J]. Medical Care, 22:543-552.

Liu G, Wu H, Sun L, et al., 2012. Chinese valuation of EQ-5D health states with the time trade-off method [J]. Value in Health, 15:A650.

Li L, Fu A Z, 2009. Some methodological issues with the analysis of preference-based EQ-5D index score [J]. Health Services and Outcomes Research Methodology, 9:162-176.

Longworth L, Bryan S, 2003. An empirical comparison of EQ-5D and SF-6D in liver transplant [J]. Health Economics, 12:1061-1067.

Luo N (a), Chew L H, Fong K Y, et al., 2003. Do English and Chinese EQ-5D versions demonstrate measurement equivalence? An exploratory study [J]. Health and Quality of Life Outcomes, 1:7.

Luo N (b), Chew L H, Fong K Y, et al., 2003. Validity and reliability of the EQ-5D self-report questionnaire in English-speaking Asian patients with rheumatic diseases in Singapore [J]. Quality of Life Research, 12: 87–92.

Luo N (c), Chew L H, Fong K Y, et al., 2003 Validity and reliability of the EQ-5D self-report questionnaire in Chinese-speaking Asian patients with rheumatic diseases in Singapore [J]. Annals Academy of Medicine Singapore, 32:685–690.

Luo N, Wang Q, Feen D, et al., 2007. Measuring health preferences for Health Utilities Index Mark 3 health states: a study of feasibility and preference differences among ethnic groups in Singapore [J]. Medical Decision Making, 27:61–70.

Luo N, Johnson J A, Shaw J W, et al., 2007. A comparison of EQ-5D index scores derived from the US and UK population-based scoring functions [J]. Medical Decision Making, 27:321–326.

Luo N, Low S, Lau P N, et al., 2009. Is EQ-5D a valid quality of life instrument in patients with Parkinson's disease? A study in Singapore [J]. Annals Academy of Medicine Singapore, 38: 521–528.

Luo N, Johnson J A, Shaw J W, et al., 2009. Relative efficiency of the EQ-5D, HUI2, and HUI3 index scores in measuring health burden of chronic medical conditions in a population health survey in the United States [J]. Medical Care, 47:53–60.

Luo N, Ko Y, Johnson J A, et al., 2009. The association of survey language (Spanish vs. English) with Health Utilities Index and EQ-5D index scores in a United States population sample [J]. Quality of Life Research, 18: 1377–1385.

Luo N, Li M, Elly A, et al., 2013. The effects of lead time and visual aids in TTO valuations: a study of the EQ-VT framework [J]. The European Journal of Health Economics, 14:S15–24.

Mann R, Brazier J, Tsuchiya A, 2009. A comparison of patient and general population weightings of EQ-5D dimensions [J]. Health Economics, 18:

References

363-372.

Marra C A, Woolcott J C, Kopec J A, et al., 2005. A comparison of generic, indirect utility measures (the HUI2, HUI3, SF-6D, and the EQ-5D) and disease-specific instruments (the RAQoL and the HAQ) in rheumatoid arthritis [J]. Social Science & Medicine, 60:1571-1582.

McDnough C M, Tosteson A N A, 2007. Measuring preferences for Cost-utility Analysis: How choice of method may influence decision-making [J]. Pharmacoeconomics, 25:93-106.

McFadden D, 1986. The choice theory approach to market research [J]. Marketing Science, 5:275-279.

McTaggart-Cowan H M, Marra C A, Yang Y, et al., 2008. The validity of generic and condition-specific preference-based instruments: the ability to discriminate asthma control status [J]. Quality of Life Research, 17: 453-462.

National Institute for Health and Clinical Excellence, 2012. Guide to the methods of technology appraisal [EB/OL]. Available from: http://www.nice.org.uk/niceMedia/pdf/TAP_Methods.pdf.

National Institute for Health and Clinical Excellence, 2013. NICE DSU technical support document 10: the use of mapping methods to estimate health state utility values [EB/OL]. Available from: http://www.nicedsu.org.uk/TSD%2010%20mapping%20FINAL.pdf.

Norman R, Cronin P, Viney R, et al., 2009. International comparisons in valuing EQ-5D health states: a review and analysis [J]. Value in Health, 12:1194-1200.

Nord E, 1995. The person-trade-off approach to valuing health care programs [J]. Medical Decision Making, 15:201-2088.

Nunnally J C, Bernstein I H, 1994. Psychometric Theory (3rd ed.) [M]. New York: McGraw-Hill.

Oppe M, Devlin N, van Hout B, et al., 2012. EuroQol Group's international protocol for the valuation of the EQ-5D-5L [R]. Proceedings of the 29th

EuroQol Plenary Meeting, September 13-15, 2012, The Doelen Convert and Congress Hall, Rotterdam, The Netherlands.

Pakir A, 1999. Bilingual education with English as an official language: Sociocultural implications [M]. In: Alatis JE, Tan AH. eds., Georgetown University Round Table on Languages and Linguistics. Washington DC: Georgetown University Press.

Patrick D L, Erickson P, 1993. Health status and health policy: Allocating resources to health care [M]. New York: Oxford University Press.

Petrou S, Hockley C, 2005. An investigation into the empirical validity of the EQ-5D and SF-6D based on hypothetical preferences in a general population [J]. Health Economics, 14:1169-1189.

Pickard S A, Tawk R, Shaw J W, 2013. The effect of chronic conditions on stated preferences for health [J]. The European Journal of Health Economics, 14:697-702.

Pickard A S, Wang Z, Walton S M, et al., 2005. Are decisions using cost-utility analyses robust to choice of SF-36/SF-12 preference-based algorithm? [J]. Health and Quality of Life Outcomes, 3:11.

Ramsey J B, 1969. Tests for specification errors in classical linear least squares regression models [J]. Journal of The Royal Statistical Society Series B-Statistical Methodology, 31:350-371.

Ratcliffe J, Brazier J, Palfreyman S, et al., 2007. A comparison of patient and population values for health states in varicose veins patients [J]. Health Economics, 16:395-405.

Revicki D A, Leidy N K, Brennan-Diemer, et al., 1998. Integrating patients' preferences into health outcomes assessment: the multi-attribute asthma symptom utility index [J]. Chest, 114:998-1007.

Revicki D, Margolis M, Thompson C, et al., 2011. Major symptom score for patients with acute rhinosinusitis [J]. American Journal of Rhinology & Allergy, 25:99-106.

Roberts B, Browne J, Ocaka K F, et al., 2008. The reliability and validity of the SF-8 with a conflict-affected population in northern Uganda [J]. Health and Quality of Life Outcomes, 6:108.

Robinson A, Spencer A, 2006. Exploring challenges to TTO utilities: valuing states worse than dead [J]. Health Economics, 15:393-402.

Rowen D, Brazier J, Roberts J, 2009. Mapping SF-36 onto the EQ-5D index: how reliable is the relationship? [J]. Health and Quality of Life Outcomes, 7:27.

Rutten-van Molken M P, Bakker C H, van Doorslaer EK, et al., 1995. Methodological issues of patient utility measurement: experience from two clinical trials [J]. Medical Care, 33:922-937.

Sackett D L, Torrance G W, 1978. The utility of different health states as perceived by the general public [J]. Journal Chronic Diseases, 31:697-704.

Samuelsen C H, Augestad L A, Stavem K, et al., 2012. Anchoring effects in the lead-time time trade-off [R]. In: Proceedings of the 29th EuroQol Plenary Meeting, September 13-15, 2012. The Doelen Concert and Congress Hall, Rotterdam, the Netherlands.

Sengupta N, Nichol M B, Wu J, et al., 2004. Mapping the SF-12 to the HUI3 and VAS in a managed care population [J]. Medical Care, 42: 927-937.

Shannon C E, 1948. A mathematical theory of communication [J]. Bell Systems Technical Journal, 27:379-423.

Shaw J W, Johnson J A, Coons S J, 2007. US valuation of the EQ-5D health states: development and testing of the D1 valuation model [J]. Medical Care, 45:238-244.

Shapiro S S, Wilk M B, 1965. An analysis of variance test for normality (complete samples) [J]. Biometrika, 52:591-611.

Silvey S D, 1959. The lagrangian multiplier test [J]. Annals of The Institute of Statistical Mathematics, 30:389-407.

Singapore Department of Statistics, 2013. Census of population 2010: statistical release 1 on demographic characteristics, education, language and religion [R/OL]. Available from: http://www.singstat.gov.sg/news/news/press12012011.pdf.

Stalmeier P F, Lamers L M, Busschbach J J, et al., 2007. On the assessment of preferences for health and duration: maximal endurable time and better than dead preferences [J]. Medical care, 45:835-841.

Streiner D L, Norman G W, 1995. Selecting the items [M]. In: Streiner D L, Norman G W, eds. Health Measurement Scales: A Practical Guide to Their Development and Use. Oxford: Oxford University Press, 39-53.

Suarez Almazor M E, Conner Spady B, 2001. Rating of arthritis health states by patients, physicians, and the general public. Implications for cost-utility analyses [J]. Journal Rheumatology, 28:648-656.

Sugimoto M, Takegami M, Suzukamo Y, et al., 2008. Health-related quality of life in Japanese men with localized prostate cancer: assessment with the SF-8 [J]. International Journal of Urology, 15:524-528.

Sullivan P W, Ghushchyan V, 2006. Mapping the EQ-5D Index from the SF-12: US general population preferences in a nationally representative sample [J]. Medical Decision Making, 26:401-409.

Thumboo J, Fong K Y, Machin D, et al., 2001. A community-based study of scaling assumptions and construct validity of the English (UK) and Chinese (HK) SF-36 in Singapore [J]. Quality of Life Research, 10:175-188.

Thurstong L L, 1927 A law of comparative judgment [J]. Psychological Review, 34:273-286.

Tongsiri S, Cairns J, 2011 Estimating population-based values for EQ-5D health states in Thailand [J]. Value in Health, 14:1142-1145.

Torrance G W, Thomas W H, Sackett D L, 1972. A utility maximization model for evaluation of health care programs [J]. Health Services Research, 7:118-133.

Torrance G W, 1986. Measurement of health state utilities for economic appraisal [J]. Journal of Health Economics, 5:1-30.

Torrance G W, 1987. Utility approach to measuring health-related quality of life [J]. Journal Chronic Diseases, 40:593-603.

Torrance G W, Feeny D, 1989. Utilities and quality-adjusted life years [J]. International Journal of Technology Assessment in Health Care, 5:559-575.

Torrance G W, Furlong W, Feeny D, et al., 1995. Multi-attribute preference functions: health utilities index [J]. Pharmacoeconomics, 7:503-520.

Treadwell J R, Lenert L A, 1999. Health values and prospect theory [J]. Medical Decision Making, 19:344-352.

Tsuchiya A, Ikeda S, Ikegami N, et al., 2002. Estimating an EQ-5D population value set: the case of Japan [J]. Health Economics, 11:341-353.

Ulber P A, Richardson J, Menzel P, 2000. Societal value, the person trade-off, and the dilemma of whose values to measure for cost-effectiveness analysis [J]. Health Economics, 9:127-136.

Ulber P A, Loewenstein G, Jepson C, 2003. Whose quality of life? A commentary exploring discrepancies between health state evaluations of patients and the general public [J]. Quality of Life Research, 12:599-607.

Von Neumann J, Morgenstern O, 1953. Theory of games and economic behavior [M]. New York: Wiley.

Walters S, Brazier J E, 2005. Comparison of the minimally important difference for two health state utility measures: EQ-5D and SF-6D [J]. Quality of Life Research, 14:1523-1532.

Wang P, Thumboo J, Lim Y W, et al., 2013. Valuation of EQ-5D-3L health states in Singapore [J]. Value in Health — Manuscript ID ViH-08-2013-0317-OM.

Wang Q, Furlong W, Feeny D, et al., 2002. How robust is the Health Utilities Index Mark 2 utility function? [J]. Medical Decision Making, 22:350-358.

Wang Y T, Lim H Y, Tai D, et al., 2012. The impact of irritable bowel syndrome on health-related quality of life: a Singapore perspective [J].

BMC Gastroenterol, 12: 104.

Ware J E., Snow K K., Kosinski M, et al., 1993. SF-36 health survey: Manual & interpretation guide [R]. Boston, MA: The Health Institute, New England Medical Centre.

Ware J E, Kosinski M, Keller S, 1996. A 12-item short-form health survey: Construction of scales and preliminary tests of reliability and validity [J]. Medical Care, 34:220-233.

Ware J E, Kosinski M, Dewey J E, et al., 2001. How to score and interpret single-item health status measures: A manual for users of the SF-8 health survey [R]. Lincoln RI: QualityMetric Incorporated.

Wee H L, Li S C, Xie F, et al., 2006. Are Asians comfortable with discussing death in health valuation studies? A study in multi-ethnic Singapore [J]. Health and Quality of Life Outcomes, 4:93.

Wee H L, Li S C, Xie F, et al., 2008. Validity, feasibility and acceptability of time trade-off and standard gamble assessments in health valuation studies: a study in a multiethnic Asian population in Singapore [J]. Value in Health, 11(Suppl 1):S3-10. Doi: 10.1111/j.1524-4733.2008.00361.x.

Wee H L, Wu Y, Thumboo J, et al., 2010. Association of body mass index with Short-form 36 physical and mental component summary scores in a multiethnic Asian population [J]. International Journal of Obesity, 34: 1034-1043.

Wittenberg E, Winer E P, Weeks J C, 2005. Patient utilities for advanced cancer: effect of current health on values [J]. Medical Care, 43:173-181.

Wittrup-Jensen K U, Lauridsen J T, Gudex C, et al., 2002. Estimating Danish EQ-5D tariffs using the time trade-off (TTO) and visual analogue scale (VAS) methods [R]. In: Norinder AL, Pedersen KM, ROOS P, editors. Proceedings of the 18th Plenary Meeting of the EuroQol Group, 2001; Copenhagen, Denmark. Lund, Sweden: Swedish Institute for Health Economics, 257-292.

World Health Organization, 2003. World Health Report 2010 [R]. Health insurance systems in China: A briefing note. Available from: http://www.who.int/healthsystems/topics/financing/healthreport/37ChinaB_YFINAL.pdf.

Yang Y, Brazier J E, Tsuchyia A, et al., 2009. Estimating a preference-based index from the Overactive Bladder Questionnaire [J]. Value in Health, 12:159-166.

Yusof F A, Goh A, Azmi S, 2012. Estimating an EQ-5D value set for Malaysia using time trade-off and visual analogue scale methods [J]. Value in Health, 15:S85-90.

Zhang X H, Li S C, Fong K Y, et al., 2009. The impact of health literacy on health-related quality of life (HRQoL) and utility assessment among patients with rheumatic diseases [J]. Value in Health, 12:S106-109.

Zhao F L, Yue M, Yang H, et al., 2010. Validation and comparison of EuroQol and short-form 6D in chronic prostatitis patients [J]. Value in Health, 13:649-656.

Zethraeus N, Johannesson M A, 1999. Comparison of patient and social tariff values derived from the time trade-off method [J]. Health Economics, 8:541-545.

图书在版编目(CIP)数据

测量健康效用以用于成本效用分析 = Measuring Health-State Utilities for Cost-Utility Analysis:英文/王沛著. —上海:复旦大学出版社,2020.11
ISBN 978-7-309-15370-5

Ⅰ.①测… Ⅱ.①王… Ⅲ.①健康状况-卫生经济学-研究-英文 Ⅳ.①R194.3

中国版本图书馆 CIP 数据核字(2020)第 203240 号

Measuring Health-State Utilities for Cost-Utility Analysis
测量健康效用以用于成本效用分析
王　沛　著
责任编辑/高　辉

复旦大学出版社有限公司出版发行
上海市国权路 579 号　邮编:200433
网址:fupnet@fudanpress.com　http://www.fudanpress.com
门市零售:86-21-65102580　团体订购:86-21-65104505
外埠邮购:86-21-65642846　出版部电话:86-21-65642845
江苏凤凰数码印务有限公司

开本 787×1092　1/16　印张 8　字数 131 千
2020 年 11 月第 1 版第 1 次印刷

ISBN 978-7-309-15370-5/R·1843
定价:38.00 元

如有印装质量问题,请向复旦大学出版社有限公司出版部调换。
版权所有　侵权必究